My dear friend

Love you with all my
heart.

Enjoy

Bernadette

Raw

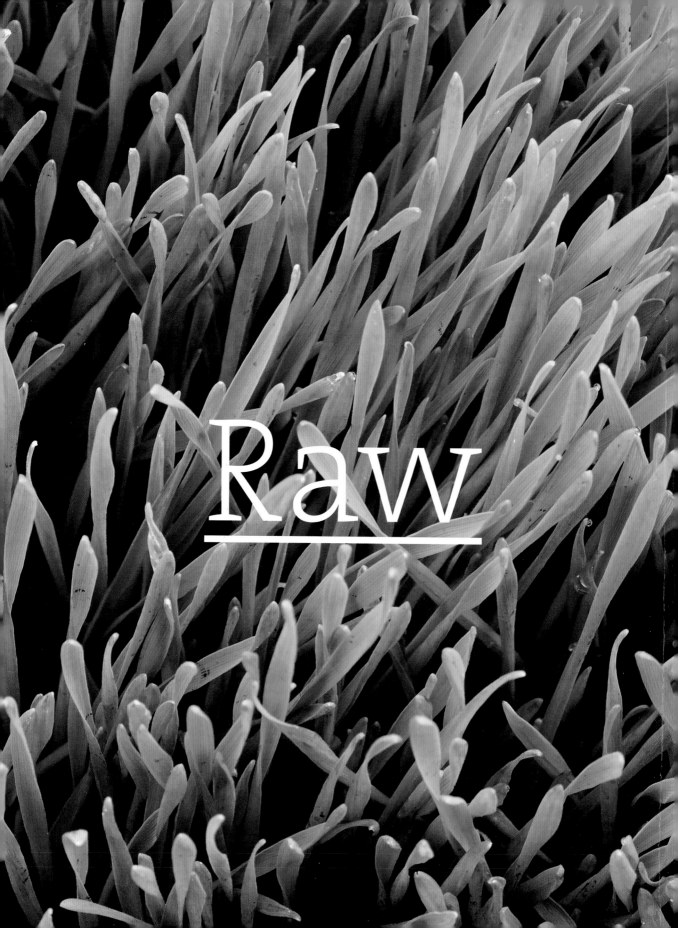

Raw

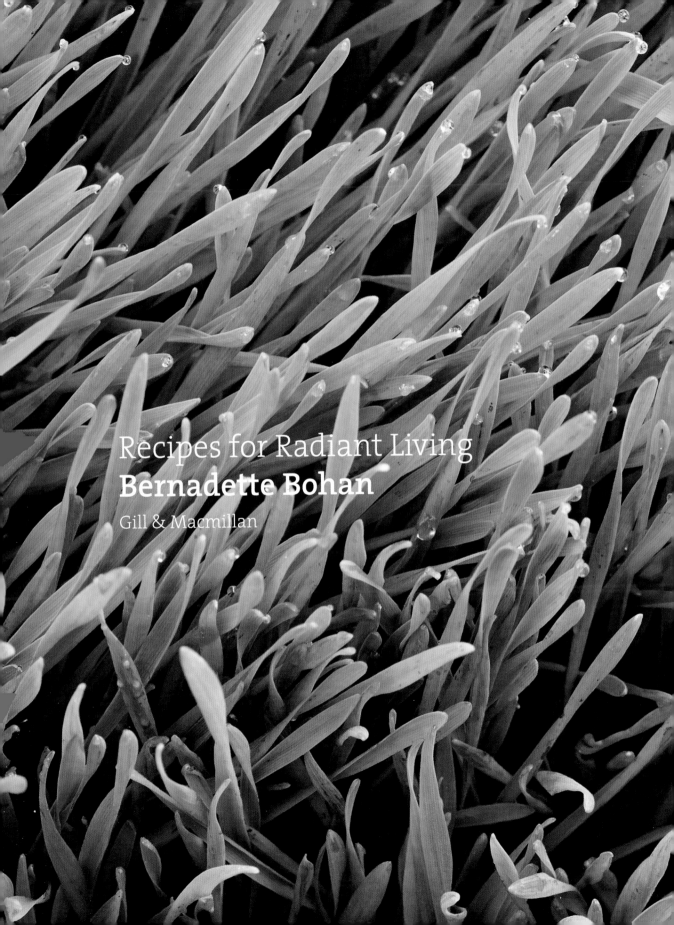

Recipes for Radiant Living
Bernadette Bohan

Gill & Macmillan

Gill & Macmillan

Hume Avenue
Park West
Dublin 12
www.gillmacmillanbooks.ie

© Bernadette Bohan 2015

978 07171 6603 9

Design by www.grahamthew.com
Photography by Neil Hurley
Photos on pp. vi, xii, 5, 23, 119, 190 © Barry McCall
Food styling by Zita Fox
Indexed by Eileen O'Neill
Printed by Printer Trento Srl, Italy

This book is typeset in 10pt The Serif on 13pt.

The paper used in this book comes from the wood pulp
of managed forests. For every tree felled, at least one
tree is planted, thereby renewing natural resources.

A CIP catalogue record for this book is available from
the British Library.

Note from the publisher

This book is written as a
source of information only and
is not intended to be taken as a
replacement for medical advice.
A qualified medical practitioner
should always be consulted before
beginning any new diet, exercise or
health plan.

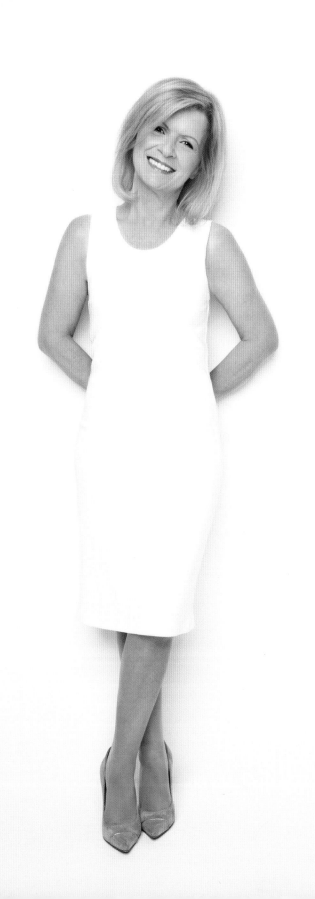

About the author

Bernadette Bohan is an ordinary woman whose life was turned upside down by two different types of cancer. She learned the value of her health the hard way, but she recovered and now feels healthier than ever.

In order to help herself through cancer treatment, Bernadette focused all her energy on getting informed about health. After meeting Dr Brian Clement from the Hippocrates Institute in Florida at a seminar, she decided to adopt the Hippocrates programme.

Firmly rooted in science, it is based on the principle that a nutrient-dense, primarily plant-based diet can lower the risk of chronic diseases, such as heart disease, diabetes and cancer, and can help us to live longer, vibrant and energetic lives.

Following the programme changed Bernadette's health for the better and she became passionate about sharing the benefits of her positive, healthy form of eating. She developed her own programme for diet and lifestyle change, which has helped thousands of people to get back to better health. For more information, visit her website: www.changesimply.com.

Bernadette is a 60-year-old mother of three who lives in Malahide, Co. Dublin, with her husband.

Heartfelt thanks to:

The love of my life, my hubby Ger. You are
a guiding light in my life. My life with you,
Richard, Sarah and Julie has been my greatest
joy. Thank you for all you do.

My taste-testing buddy, Julie, for your love,
patience, and all the sampling of recipes.

Deirdre Nolan, Teresa Daly and Catherine Gough
from Gill & Macmillan for your invaluable
experience and expertise. What a great team
you make. I feel blessed to work with you.

My good friends Geraldine, Derek, Jasmin,
Imelda and my two sisters, Deirdre and Aquinas,
for your love and encouragement.

Neil Hurley, for your attention to detail and that
bit of magic.

Zita Fox, you truly are a fox in the kitchen.

To all my readers, students and Facebook fans –
without you this book would not be possible. I wish
I could thank all of you personally.

Please know that all your efforts will help those
who are trying to improve their health.

Contents

Hot & Cold Soups & Appetizers 69

Raw & Comfort Dishes 87

Fresh Salads & Sides 115

Healthy, Nutritious Snacks & Dips

Yummy Treats & Sweets

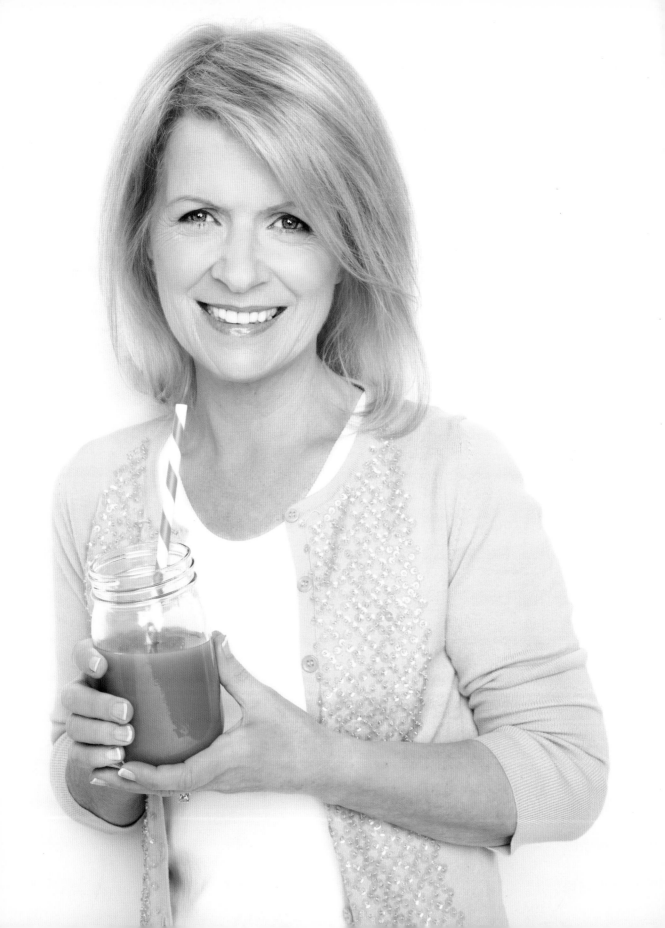

INTRODUCTION

FIFTEEN YEARS AGO life dealt me a severe blow: I was diagnosed with cancer for a second time. It was a final wake-up call. It made me focus, and prompted me to take massive action to change my lifestyle – no buts and no excuses. I now had the motivation, desire and willpower, but required the knowledge. Common sense told me that food must play an important role in health and healing. Food can be so powerful. We can easily see and feel the detrimental effects food can have on our bodies through weight and even sickness when our diet is poor. Instinctively we all know how well we feel when we eat healthily. Food keeps us alive from the cradle to the grave. So I made it my business to find out what foods make the body function correctly. Looking back, I honestly thought I was leading a healthy lifestyle; I ate fruit and veg every day, never smoked and hardly drank apart from a glass of wine with my meals. Oh yes, I was one of the 'a little bit of what you fancy will do no harm' brigade. But here I was facing cancer for a second time in 12 years. It was time to wake up and up my game.

Those of you who have read my previous books will have shared my journey. I devoured books, attended seminars and lectures, often traveling abroad trying to make sense of it all. The process was long and piecing the information together was at times arduous, particularly when the information was contradictory. It was during this period that I promised myself I would do my best to help others in a similar position in the future. I believe the most important decision you can make is to take control of your health. When you spend time preparing the foods that fuel your body, you are opening the door to real health. Most people tell me that making changes to healthier foods seems overwhelming as they are so used to 'normal' food, but believe me, if I can do it, so can you.

With this heavenly selection of delicious recipes for every occasion, you too can enjoy fabulous-tasting food that will improve your health. It's vitally important to sustain health and well-being, and yes, I understand it can be difficult if you have a busy and stressful life, especially if work and family commitments consume every moment of your day. Sometimes, no matter how much you desire a slim body, lasting energy levels or improved health, you may still find it difficult to shift your comfort zone and go for the healthy option. Although this can be frustrating, the consequences of pre-packaged sambos, ready-to-cook, ready-to-heat and ready-to-eat meals makes them definitely not the right option.

Our bodies are amazing machines. At the core of the machine is the most powerful tool we have, our immune system. The immune system, when working efficiently, will protect us and keep us healthy. But there is a deal of sorts: for it to look after us, we must look after it. How do we do this? Well, like every Irish mother knows, when you love someone, you feed them well. However ,with our immune system, it's not with comfort food. No, this baby needs fresh, plant-based nutrients to fuel it properly. Actually, come to think of it don't all mothers tell their kids to 'eat your greens'?

I know many people have a difficult time accepting that food can heal, but when you speak with people who have healed from advanced cancer without treatments you will have no trouble accepting the miraculous healing powers of nature's bounty. Meeting these people changed my whole perception of food and its ability to heal, it has been one of the key factors in making me move to a raw, living food diet. It was not just these amazing people who convinced me, let's not forget all the clinical research that has scientifically validated that there are elements in plant-based foods that literally search out, attack and destroy viruses, bacteria and cancers.

Maybe you really want to eat a healthier diet but have preconceived ideas that it is tasteless, boring or time-consuming. I promise once you taste how delicious these recipes are, it will dispel any previous notions you may have had about eating healthily. As you will see from the mouth-watering photography in this book, healthy eating is not a punishment or living on lettuce leaves and carrot sticks.

So let's look briefly at where we are coming from, before looking forward to where we need to go. Many diets predominantly contain meat, fish, chicken and dairy. Snacks, potato crisps, sugary soft drinks, processed foods with high levels of sugar and salt are regular items in the average shopping basket. Now there is little doubt, even among the most sceptical, that these foods are at best of little benefit to the immune system. It does not take a scientist to figure that out. List each off and think of the disease: it could be heart problems, cancer, arthritis, diabetes and, of course, extra weight. I realise that I may have listed some of your favourite things in the whole world and just about now you are closing the book. Please don't, your health and well-being are just too important.

The misconception is that moving from 'normal' foods can be a challenge. Sugar and salt are both highly addictive, and by and large it is this kind of addiction that keeps us in the cycle of feasting, dieting and at times feeling guilty or even depressed about our lack of control over what we eat.

So here's the deal: we will not focus on what you cannot eat or should not eat. Instead, we will focus on what you can and should eat. Through this book you will see that the transformation is not about denial, but about the feast of delicious meals and recipes that you can start eating this evening.

While teaching over the last 15 years I have seen a dramatic shift in the public's attitude to the role that diet and lifestyles play in promoting overall health. This shift in attitude has paved the way for more and more people to focus on attaining good health. So many of our television programmes now focus on the advantages of changing to a healthier lifestyle, while others focus on the increasing difficulties we face when we find ourselves on the endless conveyer belt of drugs and hospital waiting lists. There has never been a time when the old saying 'prevention is better than cure' has been so pertinent.

As I travel around the world giving seminars and workshops, I am inundated with stories that are a testament to the power of living food as medicine. My mission is to inspire you to make simple changes that will improve your health in a practical, easy and tasty way. I hope these nourishing recipes will soon form a central part of your weekly meals. Making food tasty will fast-track the switch to living on raw foods, and I have found it is the most influential way of creating lasting change. Ask my family – the toughest audience of all.

So why raw? Well, throughout the book I will explain, as we go through the recipes step by step, the advantages and benefits of the foods I use. How eating live-enzyme-rich foods we can combat everything from high cholesterol, a myriad of digestive issues and even cancer itself. I will tell you how fresh juices and veggies can provide you with all the calcium you need, something that many believe is only achievable through consuming vast amounts of dairy or calcium supplements, and how we can have the protein levels of the world's top athletes and sportspeople by eating plant-based foods.

Shortly after I started juicing fruits and vegetables and added a lot more raw foods into my diet, I saw real results. My health improved greatly, my painful arthritis disappeared, I gave up wearing my reading glasses and, as an added bonus, my spare tyre melted away – and all of these changes have remained constant ever since. The results of these simple steps sparked a true life change that altered my whole perception of cooked and raw foods. Thankfully, I am now healthier and slimmer without dieting.

The physical improvements will be your best incentive. Your health and vitality will be an advertisement for this lifestyle; you will look the picture of health. As you become more nourished by raw, living foods, you will lose the intensity of cravings. Those extra pounds will simply melt away and you won't need to pay attention to expanding waistlines. Raw, living foods do not cause the body to gain weight because you are eating foods in their natural state with all of their enzymes intact. Enzymes help us assimilate and digest foods properly.

Counting calories – a thing of the past? Never! Oh yes, definitely a thing of the past.

Rather than thinking of healthy foods in terms of restriction and deprivation, think about enjoying a thirst-quenching juice, a warm nourishing soup on a cold evening, a yummy spicy curry, pizza, pasta, cookies or a slice of delicious cheesecake all made with wholesome ingredients. How delicious does that sound? Trust me, they taste just as good as they sound.

Eating raw, living foods will inject vitality into your life, it has certainly brought my health to a different level. It has changed my life immeasurably and that is why I feel so passionate to share with you how to enjoy this positive healthy form of eating. With extraordinary visual appeal, these foods not only look and taste delicious but will help fulfil your body's crucial need for nutrients. I have included a selection of staple family favourites as well as a myriad of refreshing new choices that will help you transform fruits and vegetables into fantastic dishes that will satisfy even a fussy palate.

The recipes in this book will help you create a lifestyle that is sustainable, which will ultimately lead to a healthier, happier you. Remember: you are the one who can make the biggest impact on your own health. *You* get to choose. But don't take my word for it. Just look at the yummy, nutritious food. And as good as the dishes look, they taste even better. They are delicious, the majority are raw, and you can prepare these tried and tested dishes in your own home.

Are you ready to join me and take a culinary excursion into the wonderful world of raw foods?

With love,
Bernadette

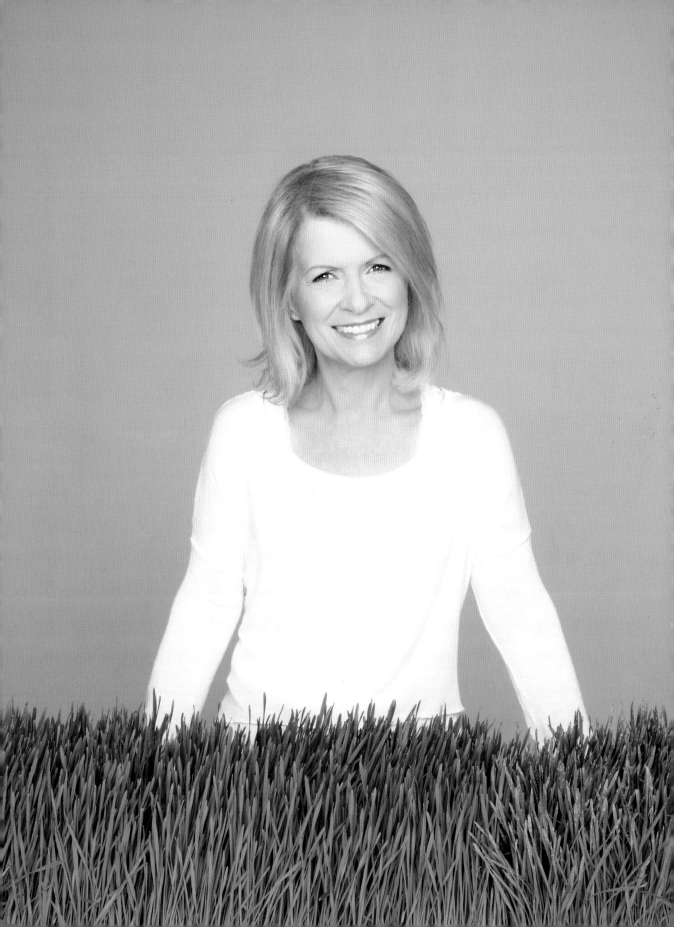

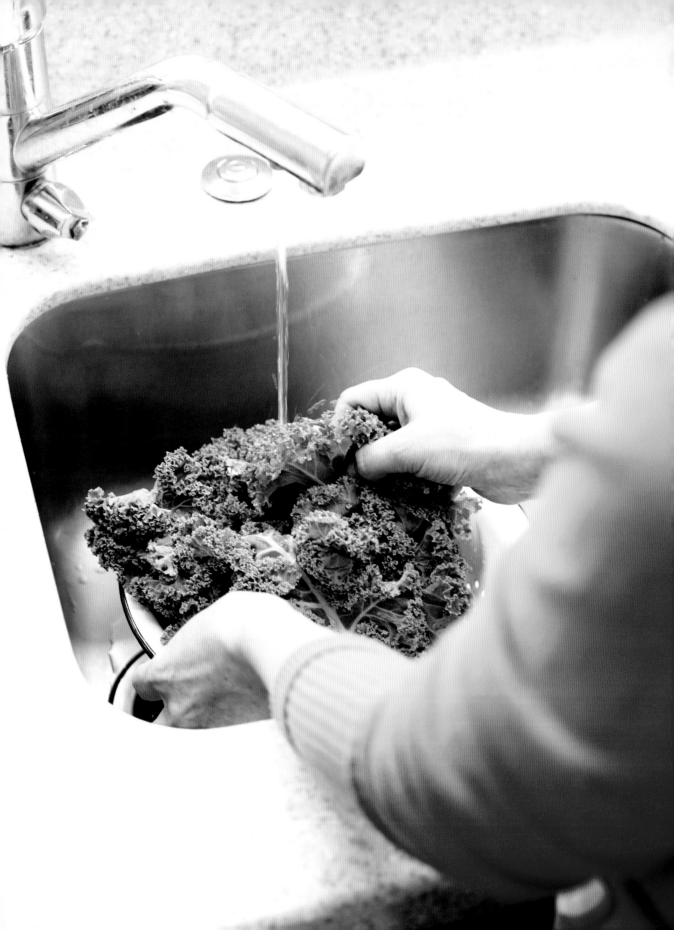

WHAT ARE RAW, LIVING FOODS?

'Dead or Live'

The logic underpinning the raw, living foods diet is pretty much common sense. Think of it in terms of 'live foods' or 'dead foods'. Live foods are foods that have not been denatured by heat, and as such their nutrients and enzymes remain intact. Eating raw, living foods has become the 'in' thing among consumers who are concerned about the foods they eat. Naturally, live foods nourish your body more than dead foods.

It's wonderful to see people get back to some grass-roots solutions to protect their health. It's not surprising that people make the switch, when you consider that many of the foods we eat today are often far removed from their original natural state, and can be highly processed, laden with sugars, additives and preservatives, all of which have negative effects on our health. The scandals in the food chain over the last few years have made us think twice about the foods we eat. Foods we blindly trusted and thought were good for us, we subsequently found are detrimental to our health. Yet a few years ago, we ate and gave them to our children in abundance.

Most of us have tunnel vision when it comes to food, but the fact is that many of the foods that are eaten today not only lack nourishment but also contain harmful ingredients. Some foods labelled as being the 'healthy option', 'healthy choice' or 'healthy alternative' should possibly be better labelled 'buyer beware'. Let's not beat about the bush here: the desire for profit is the motivating force behind much of the food that is available for sale, as it is based on economics and not health. By eating living foods, you won't need to waste time checking out the hidden ingredients in these not-so-healthy products.

Thankfully, consumers are waking up to the fact that food manufacturers are now selling ready-meals in the guise of health foods. If you were to check your kitchen cupboards or freezer, how much of that food have you bought because of convenience, and how much has been bought to nourish your body?

If you really want to recharge your batteries, eat more raw, living food. Heating your food is not as good for your health because cooked food causes an inflammatory response in the body called leukocytosis (elevated number of white cells in the blood). Leukocytes play an important role in the body's immune system to fight against infections. When food is heated above 40 degrees Celsius, its molecular structure changes: oils turn carcinogenic and proteins, vitamins and live enzymes are destroyed in the cooking process. The Max Planck Institute in Leipzig found that cooking denatures proteins, which means that our bodies have to work harder to assimilate these dead foods. Because the beneficial enzymes have been destroyed by cooking, the food is difficult to digest and provides very little nourishment.

When foods are not cooked, their nutrients remain intact and, more significantly, live enzymes – the most important part of our foods – are not destroyed. All cellular activity of life depends on enzymes, so much so that without them, there would be no life. Enzymes such as amylase, protease and lipase are necessary for digestion. Enzymes stimulate the body's killer T-cells to destroy cancer cells. Enzymes enhance longevity significantly, as they slow down free-radical damage. This is another great reason to eat more raw, living foods. It is definitely worth making the effort to prepare foods that will provide your body with much more nutrition.

As the saying goes, it's not the food in your life, but the life in your food that nourishes your body.

Dead food

You cannot expect to thrive on the lifeless energy of dead foods. Food gives us energy, but when we consume 'dead' foods we feel lethargic and heavy. Many of the valuable nutrients that are needed for repairing and rebuilding our cells are heat sensitive. Cooking destroys enzymes and forces the body to produce more of its own enzymes, which are secreted by our pancreas, and this leaves little left over to fight off disease. Enzyme depletion has been associated with arthritis, allergies, cancer and cardiovascular disease.

On average the cooking process destroys:

- 50 per cent of the minerals
- 75 per cent of the vitamins
- 100 per cent of the enzymes, hormones, oxygen and phytonutrients.

Take minerals as an example – they are more abundant in raw plant foods. Plants pick up 70 to 80 different minerals from the soil and make them available to us. This is why your mother always told you to eat your greens. When we heat these, 50 per cent of their valuable nutrients are lost. Foods that are stripped of nutrients will not fuel the cells of your body. Rather, they will leave you with an exhausted immune system.

Living on raw, live foods is a much healthier option than one based on cooked foods. If you are not inclined to give up your cooked meals, you could always try my dehydrated recipes. These taste great and alter the texture a little to make them more like cooked foods. The lower temperature preserves the nutrients and gives you yummy, tasty meals. If you are starting out, aim to have 50 per cent of your daily foods raw and 50 per cent cooked, and gradually work your way up to 80 per cent raw and 20 per cent cooked. Add sprouts to your meals or salads and they will supply vital nutrients to your daily diet. If you make it all the way to 100 per cent, it would be amazing for your health. This recipe book will help you achieve your health goals. It's a recipe book that'll get you eating healthier and better than ever, and I am so passionate about the benefits of eating raw foods that I absolutely guarantee you will notice the difference.

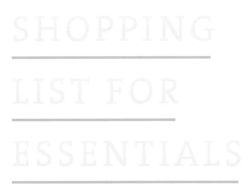

SHOPPING LIST FOR ESSENTIALS

Make a shopping list. A list can determine the foods that fill your kitchen cupboards and freezer. Never go shopping on an empty tummy or you will find yourself taking the easy options from your old habits as opposed to nutrition-based choices. We have a massive assortment of unhealthy foods at our fingertips, so remember convenience is a big selling point. They are foods for profit, not health. Stick with the list and avoid the food aisles that stock processed, sugary foods. There may be a few items below that you don't recognise, but as you become familiar with the recipes it will all start to fit together and help you to maintain a well-balanced diet.

SWEETENERS

Coconut milk, coconut cream, dried coconut, carob powder, stevia, vanilla extract, maple flavour, dried fruits, Teeccino coffee replacement.

SAVOURY SEASONING

Celery salt, paprika, cayenne pepper, pizza seasoning, oregano, basil, parsley, chipotle powder, garlic and onion powder. While fresh herbs give the nicest flavour, it is handy as a back-up to have a variety of dried ones also. Bragg Liquid Aminos is a wheat-free and salt-free liquid seasoning that contains essential amino acids.

SEAWEEDS

Kelp, nori, dulse, wakame and arame.

NUTS

Pecans, walnuts, almonds, Brazil, macadamia and pine nuts (although actually a seed). No peanuts or cashews.

VEGGIES

I could make a long list of veggies, but really just choose whatever is in season, and ideally locally grown. A few of my weekly essentials are salad leaves, avocados, onions, celery, cucumber, garlic and ginger root.

SPROUTING SEEDS

Alfalfa, broccoli, buckwheat, garlic, onion, sesame, fenugreek, pea, pumpkin and sunflower seeds.

GRAINS

Millet, buckwheat, quinoa and teff.

BEANS FOR SPROUTING

Mung, aduki, lentils and chickpeas.

You're only as good as your tools. Think health, not wealth.

Central to your raw, living foods kitchen are a few core pieces of equipment. Of course there is some initial cost, but think of this equipment as an investment in your health. If you want to maximise your chances of living a long, healthy, productive life you will need the tools to help you do so. Believe me, it is much better to increase your chances of living a healthier life than to navigate your way through health issues. Think about your health as an investment, not an expense. Investing in your health should be a priority, especially if you want to minimise the soaring cost of healthcare. If we treat our health like another expense, and fail to make it a priority, it could work out more expensive in the long run. When you care enough to invest in your health, everyone gains. It is not only good for you, but also for the health of your entire family.

The first and probably the most difficult step is knowing where to start. Here are some guidelines of the tried-and-tested equipment in my kitchen. This guide will get you started and give you the resources and guidance you need to help you spend your money wisely. Having the right tools for the job is essential to getting the right results.

Buying a juicer

Top of the list is a masticating juicer. It's so easy to implement a daily routine of juicing, all you need is just some fresh fruit and vegetables and a good juicer.

There are basically three types of juicer available. If you are inexperienced, you could spend a great deal of time deciding whether to go for a masticating juicer or the cheaper centrifugal models. Some people start out with the centrifugal juicers but then upgrade to a masticating juicer because of the drawbacks of the centrifugal models. Of course you want a good juicer at a competitive price, but don't compromise and start with a juicer that is difficult to wash, as it will put you off juicing. After the initial outlay, I am sure you will find no comparison in the quality and quantity of the juice from a masticating machine versus that of a centrifugal juicer.

Masticating juicers are not usually sold in the high street as they are a bit more of a specialty – check out the Resources section at the end of the book for suppliers.

Masticating juicers

Twin-gear masticating juicers produce the best quality juice, and cost about €500. I use my Green Star juicer not only for juicing, but also to make pizza and pie crusts, pâtés from nuts and vegetables, sauces and yummy treats. If you think a masticating juicer is out of your price range or wondering if its worth the cost, bear these few points in mind:

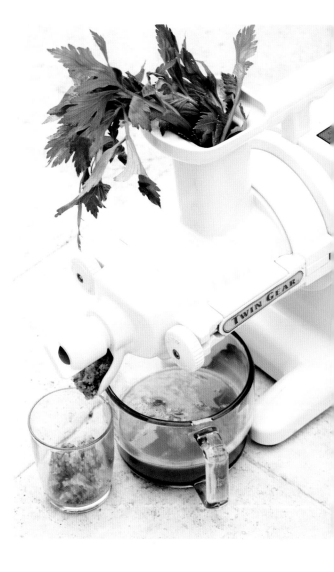

- Masticating juicers are very economical as they produce very small amounts of dry pulp, which ensures you get the best possible value – the most juice – from your produce.

- Their strong triturating and squeezing power extracts more minerals from your produce, which gives you a better quality juice. They have automatic pulp ejection, and the pulp can even be returned to the chute to extract more juice.

- They produce twice as much juice as centrifugal juicers. If you juice even four times per week (especially if it's for two or three people) the price difference between the masticating and centrifugal juicer will easily be paid in a year just from the savings on produce.

- A really important point to look out for when buying a juicer is the two gears that grind the fruit and vegetables slowly. The twin gears revolve very slowly while grinding so that no heat is produced, which means you get a superior quality juice.

- Masticating juicers are outstanding for juicing kale, parsley, chard, lettuce, turnip greens and spinach; the gears suck the leafy greens in and grind them up without clogging.

- One of the big advantages of these machines is their ability to reconstruct the water molecules in the juice. It does this by magnetically extracting minerals from fruits and vegetables through magnetic technology, which reduces oxidation of the juice. For a good quality juice, you want a juicer that oxidises the juice minimally as it's being made.

- There are single-gear masticating juicers that are cheaper (about €200–300). These juicers will do a similar job to the twin-gear juicers. If you are on a budget, the Samson 6-in-1 will do a good job. It can juice wheat grass, fruits, leafy green vegetables and herbs, which most juicers bought in the high street stores won't.

- Masticating juicers don't require any messy greasing before use, unlike other juicers.

- The tiny screen requires a bit of scrubbing, but a really handy tip is to open the nozzle at the front and pour a jug of water down the chute while the machine is running. This cleans out most of the remaining pulp and a rinse under the tap removes the rest.

- There are various accessories that are supplied with the more expensive models such as pasta- and bread-stick-makers.

Centrifugal juicers

I am not a fan of centrifugal juicers because they use the power of centrifugal force to separate the pulp from the juice; this tears up the fruits and vegetables and destroys the enzymes in the juice, the most important part. The question is why juice with a machine that produces a poor-quality juice? I can't see the sense in that. When I started juicing I made the mistake of buying a centrifugal juicer because they were cheaper and readily available.

- The high revolutions produce a poor-quality juice, which for me is a big design flaw. They mainly extract the water from the fruits and veg. If you have one of these juicers, you will notice how the juice separates.

- They are also quite wasteful of produce as they produce a lot of wet pulp, which can become very expensive, particularly if you are buying organic produce.

- The spinning, fine-mesh basket inside the machine is a pain to wash. A machine that is difficult to wash is the major reason why people who start juicing enthusiastically soon pack it in.

- The other let-down is that the appliance gets jammed and clogged easily, which is a major annoyance.

- I also question their durability. If you are juicing every day or juicing for a family, these machines can burn out easily and need replacing. I had two machines in the past that burned out, which was costly in the long term.

- Finally, centrifugal juicers won't juice wheatgrass or leafy greens. They tend to get stuck and can jam the machine. You end up stuffing in leafy greens and trying to force them through the machine.

Manual juicers

- These are very affordable; however, they are a little difficult to use and wash.

- In comparison with the electric-powered models, they are not as good at juicing fibrous veggies like carrots and celery.

- They can juice wheatgrass and leafy greens and, as a result, most people tend to buy them just for wheatgrass juicing.

- Manual juicers are handy if you are travelling, because they are lightweight and portable, which means you can make your own fresh juice wherever you go.

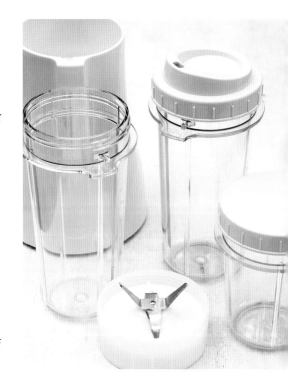

If you're serious about your health, remember: a juicer is an investment in your health and your future. Throughout the book you will find lots of deliciously healthy juice recipes to delight and turn on your palate. Happy juicing!

Smoothie-maker

A smoothie-maker makes delicious smoothies, sauces and baby foods in seconds. The big advantage of some of them is that you can drink straight from the cup, which saves on washing a cumbersome smoothie jug. With less cleaning up, you are more likely to stick with your health plan over time. Look for one that has BPA-free poly-carbonate cups that are dishwasher safe. Other features to look out for include extra compact cups that are light enough for lunch boxes, or taking a smoothie or protein drink to work, and a commuter sipping lid, which is so convenient if you drink on the run. A go-anywhere blender makes healthy living more convenient and easy.

It's ideal for a quick healthy drink in the morning if you are short on time, and it's a healthy way to start the day, and faster than preparing toast or cereal. You can make low-calorie smoothies that contain tons of great health benefits.

Dehydrator

This is a small and inexpensive drying machine that warms food slightly as it removes the moisture from fresh food without destroying the nutrients, and gives the finished dish the appearance of being cooked. A dehydrator is an excellent piece of kitchen equipment that will make crisps, snacks, biscuits, crackers and main meals. You can also make snacks from leftover produce like apples, bananas, herbs, etc. These super-healthy foods are tastier than shop-bought products and have the added advantage of being free from artificial preservatives. The snacks are great if you get the munchies while watching television or sitting at your desk and are fantastic for kids' lunchboxes.

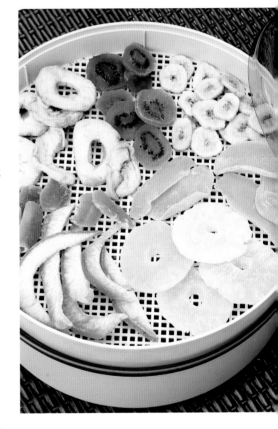

With a small investment in a dehydrator you can produce satisfying, tasty and enzyme-rich foods for yourself and your family. It's worth the investment for the crisps alone. Don't be put off by the length of time it takes to dry the foods. The time is not spent preparing the food, it's just the length of time it takes to dry it out. A dehydrator is not like an oven; there is no risk of burning the food, so you don't have to watch over it.

Dehydrators are relatively inexpensive; the Stockli dehydrator is about €150. Mine is in constant use in my kitchen, as it's simple to use and keep clean, and is very efficient. It has a variable temperature adjustment ranging between 20°C and 70°C, so you can make sure that you choose a temperature that will preserve the nutritional content of your produce. Three trays are standard, but it can be expanded to use up to ten trays. I initially bought a larger one because I do so many demonstrations, but I found it bulky and the food dried around the edges and not in the centre, which was a nuisance, so I'd definitely recommend a more compact model.

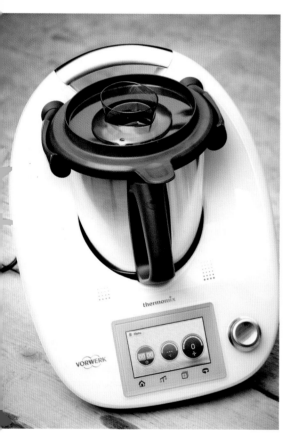

Power blender

Preparing raw sauces, dips, milks, ice-creams and cheesecakes is all about consistency, and a good power blender offers precision and consistency every time. I use a Thermomix as it has a wide bowl and detachable blades, so you can scrape out the contents of the bowl easily and avoid wastage. It's much more than a blender; in fact, it chops, stirs, kneads, emulsifies, mixes, whips, grinds, minces, grates, blends, heats, steams and even weighs food.

I find the Thermomix power blender super for grinding nuts, grains and whole foods, making favourites like almond biscuits, pie crusts, pâtés from nuts and vegetables, sauces from a vast array of ingredients, baby foods and frozen fruit desserts. The motor is really powerful and it makes light work of crushing and blending ice cubes and frozen ingredients. It takes the chore out of chopping onions, potatoes, carrots and herbs – you simply select the speed to control how coarsely or finely you want your ingredients chopped. You can even chop very small amounts of food, like a single onion, in just a few seconds. For bread-making it is superb, as the dough mode imitates the kneading action of a professional baker with an intermittent clockwise/counter-clockwise motion.

Many years of experience have taught me that if you buy cheap you buy twice. It is serious money – about €1,100 – but this labour-saving device will save you time and a ton of elbow grease. Of course you could save your money by doing these tasks yourself, but life is too short for that. If you are considering buying a power blender, I can tell you I would not trade mine for the world.

Sprouting jars

You don't need to be a keen gardener in order to grow your own sprouts. Believe me, it really is child's play. Children grow alfalfa and cress in their first year in school, so no excuses. You just soak the seeds, drain them, rinse them once a day and leave them to grow. By growing your own sprouts you are literally growing your own organic vegetables. Sprouts are very much part of my lifestyle, and I have various sprouts like alfalfa, broccoli and radish growing in jars.

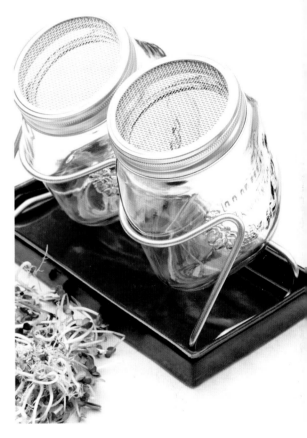

I have tried and tested many different gadgets for growing sprouts and always end up going back to the glass jar system. Why so? Well I find some of the other gadgets a pain to wash, and I am all for making life easy. The glass jars set with stainless steel rack and ceramic drip tray is a complete kit. It's easy to use and easy to wash – a big plus. I pop the jars in the dishwasher along with the mesh lids. Some of the key factors in sprouting are moisture and oxygen. Moisture activates the seeds to germinate and begin the growing process, and you need good circulation of air to produce mould-free sprouts. A good set has a stainless steel rack angled at 45 degrees, which allows better drainage and ventilation, unlike the plastic versions. They are also dishwasher safe.

Sprouting seeds and beans is inexpensive and an excellent way to ensure that you and your family have a good supply of vitamins and minerals. Sprouts are constantly growing, right up until the time of consumption. Add them to juices, soups, sandwiches, salads and main meals.

Vegetable spiraliser

This is a fab kitchen gadget for the living-food enthusiast. It's easy to use and you can make spaghetti, vegetable noodles, potato chips and shoestring potatoes, all from veggies. How cool is that?

It's a great way to jazz up a salad as it adds interesting textures. The noodles are perfect for 'stir-raws' (-fries) and salads, and the interchangeable blades can cut cucumber, carrots, sweet potato butternut squash, courgettes, radishes and apples in seconds. An easy gadget to use, you simply pop the veggies on the spikes and turn the handle to produce beautiful spaghetti, spirals or ribbons instantly. Kids love the interesting shapes and it's a great way to get them to eat more veggies.

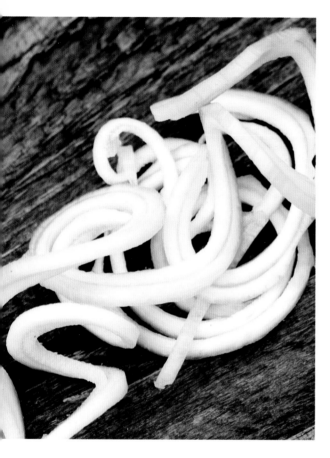

You can also create fine shoestring garnishes just like restaurant chefs and impress your dinner guests. It rinses very easily under the tap – I do this the minute I am finished, before food dries onto it. The blades and cutters are very sharp, so as with any blade, be careful.

Measuring cups and spoons

A traditional measuring set is invaluable. It's much easier to measure in cups for raw food recipes as they don't have to be so exact. They cost about €5.

Sharp knives

I am not going to harp on about sharp knives as I am sure you already know that a good set of sharp knives makes life easier in the kitchen. Enough said.

Water distiller

Clean water is essential for a healthy body. It is so easy to clean the water coming into your home, no matter what your budget. Nothing is more important for you and your family's health than clean water. Tap water contains measurable amounts of several contaminants. You may find it hard to swallow tap water when you discover it contains toxic chemicals, such as chlorine, fluoride, lead and aluminium. The problems associated with tap water have been widely publicised. A recent report from the Drinking Water Inspectorate in the UK revealed that, despite widespread purification treatments, pharmaceutical drugs are finding their way into the water supply. Another report in the US from the Environmental Protection Agency revealed that in just one single year, 2.4 billion pounds of cancer-causing materials were released into the environment and stated that much of these cancer-causing toxins and chemicals found their way into water and food supplies.

To help you evaluate the different options, I have picked an economically priced distiller, a reasonably priced reverse-osmosis system and a more up-market atmospheric purification system.

DISTILLERS

- Distillers are the most economical and effective ways to remove chemicals and purify water.
- They are simple to operate, do not require installation and are basically maintenance-free.
- The initial outlay is not expensive – around €280 – and consumption of electricity is minimal, which means you get pure water at the lowest possible cost.
- Distillers eliminate the cost and inconvenience of buying bottled mineral water.
- Distillers clean the water of 99 per cent of impurities, bacteria and chemicals.
- Distilled water produces a negative ion reaction in the system; negative ions are alkaline-forming.

VORTEX WATER REVITALIZER

- When water goes through a Vortex Water Revitalizer it is revitalised with oxygen, energy and higher frequencies that purify, sterilise and oxygenate your water back to a 'living water' state.
- The Vortex Water Revitalizer has an internal double-spiral flow form that simulates the natural movement of water in nature. When the water flows into the Vortex Revitalizer, it is being split into two parallel streams. This natural life-

forming energetic implosion process allows denatured, lifeless tap water to be brought back to its natural state and be instilled with its natural, life supporting properties. By putting water through its natural flow dynamics, water's self-cleaning, antibacterial properties are restored, it is brought to a natural pH balance, and it is naturally softened.

The three most important benefits of revitalizing your water are:

1 Your water becomes instantly absorbed by your body and tastes great.

2 Revitalised water increases the amount of dissolved oxygen in your water towards its natural level.

3 It eliminates and prevents slimy bacteria build-up.

I use a five-stage reverse osmosis system, which removes the majority of the contaminants that are found in regular drinking water. I have also attached a Vortex Water Revitalizer to the system, and the end result is pure, living water.

REVERSE OSMOSIS

This domestic drinking water system is most commonly known for its use in converting sea water into drinking water, though they are also made for both mains and well-water sources.

- A reverse-osmosis system sits under your kitchen sink. It connects to a separate tap on your sink unit, and it is also possible to connect to a refrigerator's water supply for making ice.

- It is a filtration method that removes contaminants such as chlorine, fluoride and other chemical contaminants, heavy metals, bacteria, viruses, organic compounds and even radioactive materials, which ensures about a 95 per cent purity rate for your drinking water.

- It is especially important to make sure that source water passes through a five-micron sediment filter as otherwise it can affect the taste and appearance of the water. Many of the cheaper versions only have one- or two-stage carbon filters systems; these cheap systems really only filter out large molecules from the water and don't clean the water sufficiently.

- The cost of the system supplied and fitted is usually about €400. There are cheaper systems on the internet, but keep in mind that you will have to find a plumber to fit the system. You will need an annual service to maintain it and change the replacement cartridges in the years to come. See Resources, page 194.

Besides cleaning the water in your home, a home system has much less impact on the environment than plastic water bottles, an important factor for the next generation.

ATMOSPHERIC WATER

This system uses reverse-osmosis technology but requires no water source. It creates drinking water out of the moisture in the atmosphere, which means that this type of generator extracts water from vapour in the atmosphere and converts it into pure drinking water.

- The major advantage with this system is there is no ground water contamination.
- They are a good replacement for conventional water coolers in offices as they cut down on lugging heavy water bottles about, and can be used wherever there is an electrical outlet nearby. If you buy bottled water, be aware that the plastic used to make water bottles (polyethylene terephthalate) leaches oestrogens into the water and generates 100 times the amount of toxic emissions as the same amount of glass.
- These systems dehumidify your working and living environment, and purify the air you breathe. They also eliminate over 90 per cent of airborne germs and dust found in the air.
- They are useful in locations where water is scarce or expensive.
- As a cost comparison these systems come with a sizeable up-front investment. The various models range from €1,800 to €2,000.

Drinking water has many benefits and I encourage you to drink lots of it for the sake of your health – just make sure you know its source.

Check the labels for health enhancer and immune booster recipes

The recipes are separated into two groups: health enhancer recipes and immune booster recipes. Although this book is mostly raw, I have added a few cooked dishes to help you through the transition phase. They will give you comfort, familiarity and ease your way forward.

When you are trying to change poor eating habits it helps enormously if you get your head in the right place. Your mental approach can work for you or be one of the biggest drawbacks you will face. Think about it: if your mind is constantly nagging you with the whys and wherefores, will it make for a smooth transition? There is enough research in recent years to show that negative thoughts influence the physical biology of the body. A positive, focused attitude is the key to a smooth transition, it could be just as important for the body as eating nourishing foods.

The recipes marked 'health enhancer' are for those of you who want to make some changes to improve your health but who are not facing a health challenge. They include fruits and potatoes, which are omitted from the immune booster recipes.

You don't have to change your entire diet at once, unless you want to. Drastic changes in diet are hard to stick with – you might last a week or two before you start craving all the stuff you are psychologically attached to. Cleaning out the fridge of all the familiar food you normally eat and replacing it with a field of green veggies may not be a wise move in the first week.

The easiest way to transition to better health is to transition gradually. You'll find it's not as tough as you think. These recipes will help you successfully transition to a healthier diet without starving yourself or feeling deprived. All of the immune booster recipes can also be used by those going through the transition phase.

Immune booster recipes

The 'immune booster' recipes are for those of you who want to lose weight or are facing a health challenge. Many people only change their eating habits when they are forced to because of a health issue. It's so important to eat nutritious foods when you are unwell, especially if you lose your appetite or desire to eat. This is where raw foods help, as enzymes help digest foods and are responsible for all of the work done inside our cells. As all digestion begins at a cellular level, eating enzyme-rich foods is an inexpensive, reliable way to feed your cells and rejuvenate your health.

Eating nutritious foods is a very effective way to create a body that is resistant to disease. Mother Nature has laced thousands of foods with nutrients that help keep infections and other illnesses at bay. The immune booster recipes will also help you lose unwanted weight permanently without depriving yourself.

One of my students recently lost two and a half stone in weight. She had tried all the sexy temporary diets for years but they had no lasting results. She simply made a few small changes, and she prepares all her food now herself, even though she insisted she was useless in the kitchen. Thankfully, with raw foods you don't need to be a chef. Small changes helped her break harmful habits and create better ones. What better way to improve your health and looks than with delicious nutritious foods? Foods that are rich in antioxidant and anti-inflammatory components, as well as essential enzymes, vitamins and minerals.

These immune booster recipes are a bit more hard core. I have chosen these particular recipes because they won't spike your blood sugars, and so they don't increase weight gain or encourage the growth of fungus, yeasts, parasites and cancer. The bottom line is nutrition, complemented by a good mental attitude and physical activities, which are all essential elements for those on the path to better health. Real health is more than simply taking care of the physical.

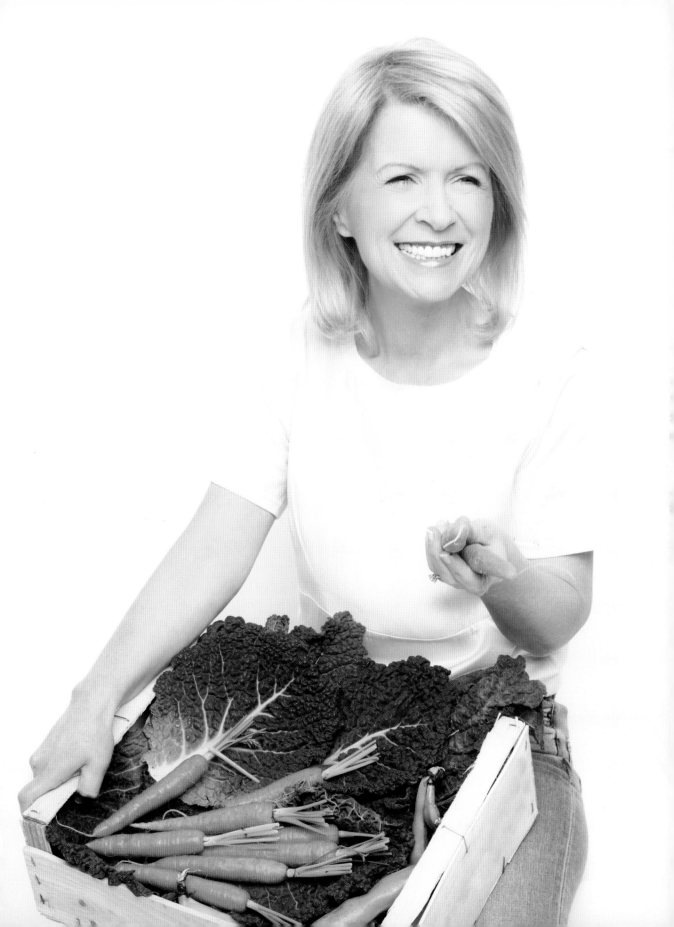

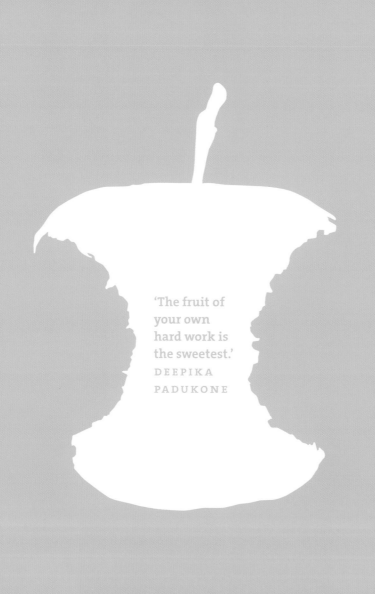

'The fruit of
your own
hard work is
the sweetest.'
DEEPIKA
PADUKONE

Nutritious, Fresh Juices & Drinks

If health, taste and simplicity are what motivate you, then your first port of call is fresh veggie juices. I cannot recommend these therapeutic juices enough. Juices will give you a new lease of life; you will immediately feel the benefits of juicing veggies because they have amazing nutritional benefits. They taste fantastic and are easily absorbed by the body. The three main reasons for juicing are hydration, cleansing and, last but not least, the flood of absorbable nutrients that heal and repair your cells.

HEALING

Let's start with the wonderful healing properties of fresh veggie juices. Notice that I have made a distinction between fruits and veggies. I am not a big fan of fruit juices, although I have added some to this book, hoping that their sweet taste will get you started. In my early days of juicing I used large amounts of apples and carrots, as carrots are rich in carotenoids such as beta-carotene. Of course my eyesight improved, as beta-carotene is fantastic at enhancing eyesight. But little did I know at that stage that carrots are also loaded with sugar (fructose). Sugars have a detrimental effect on our health – even natural sugars such as fructose. Vegetable juices are less taxing on our blood-sugar levels than fruit juices, which can spike blood sugars.

Veggie juices will boost your natural defences because they are highly concentrated forms of nutrition. Their therapeutic properties are of particular value to people fighting any kind of disease. Green juices are a major part of the Hippocrates Health programme, which I have followed now for fifteen years. If you lack energy or need a quick pick-me-up to overcome fatigue or the dreaded afternoon slump, veggie juices will recharge your batteries and give you the stamina you need; they are the perfect antidote to fatigue. They increase your intake of vital nutrients such as enzymes, phytonutrients, vitamins, minerals and amino acids. To boost energy levels and maximise your ability to fight disease go for green juices made with cucumbers, celery, kale, spinach and sprouts. You can flavour them with lemon or ginger.

HYDRATION

Staying hydrated is of major importance as our bodies' systems depend heavily on water. When you are dehydrated, your body's response is to decrease urine output in order to conserve water. Your organs cannot function well without water, so your body prioritises their needs first, compromising other bodily functions. As your body tries to prevent water loss, it extracts water from other areas: the lymphatic system (which removes toxins from the body), the blood stream (which carries oxygen around the body) and the colon (which removes waste), not to mention your skin and your joints. By drinking fresh vegetable juices, you can easily cut out empty calories from soft drinks that contain artificial sweeteners. Chemical sweeteners in diet soft drinks acidify the body and cause you to retain fluids, giving you a bloated appearance. Carbonated soft drinks contain phosphoric acid, which accelerates bone loss. Besides, think of the money you'll save on soft drinks and carton juices, which lose their beneficial enzymes in the pasteurisation process.

What better way to hydrate and increase your intake of veggies than with these delicious juices? Cucumbers are full of water – that's why they are the base of most green juices. With just two glasses of juice per day, you can hydrate your body with nourishing veggies – a much better bet than the fluoridated water that comes out of most taps. If you find drinking large amounts of water difficult, the taint of the chemicals that are added to your water might be the reason.

Two delicious juices can easily increase your fluid intake. For two 225 ml glasses of juice per day, I use 2 large cucumbers, 4 sticks of celery, a few stalks of kale and two handfuls of sprouts. If I tried to chomp my way through that lot it would take the entire afternoon, and I am not sure my teeth would stand it. Yes, I know 14 cucumbers in a week sounds like a lot of extra shopping, but don't you deserve the best? Think of all that raw liquid nutrition that will hydrate your skin and enhance your stamina and vitality. Your shopping list will change, but you will have the satisfaction of knowing that your freshly extracted juices have no artificial colourings, flavours or preservatives because you made them yourself. Remember, carbonated and carton drinks can work out to be expensive by comparison with fresh juices.

CLEANSING

Juices are a great way to stimulate better elimination of wastes and toxins and assist with the detoxification process. I can't begin to tell you the stories people tell me (well, not in a recipe book anyway) of how juicing has helped them move mountains (a bit too much information, maybe). If you want a spring clean from the inside, there is no better way to gently remove the clogged up accumulations of waste and toxins that live in our digestive tract. Believe me, when you drink a 225 ml glass of juice first thing in the morning, it will flush out your system very thoroughly and assist in the important task of cleaning out the intestines.

Veggie juices are so easy to assimilate compared to solid foods as the fibre is removed. This means the workload for our digestive system is reduced, and you can take in the fibre you need through your food throughout the rest of the day. Adding lemons to your juices for extra flavour is also beneficial, as they have many medicinal properties. Lemons are rich in vitamin C and also contain small amounts of niacin and thiamine. The vitamin C content of lemons not only helps to stave off colds, it is also very effective at cleaning the digestive tract, and great for helping us to metabolise calcium. Use the skin of lemons, too, as they are loaded with phytonutrients, but make sure the lemons are organic to avoid exposure to pesticides. I find that including the skin of the lemon gives a nice zing to various juices; I use skin, pith and even the seeds.

If you want to nurture your body with the correct fuel, age well and help your body become a picture of health, get into the juicing habit. I guarantee you will soon reap the rewards of this not-so-fruit-full diet. Sláinte!

IMMUNE-BOOSTER JUICE

IMMUNE BOOSTER

Most juices contain fruits, but it's green veggie juices that alkalise the body. When the body fluids contain too much acid, it is known as acidosis. Acidosis occurs when your kidneys and lungs can't keep your body's pH in balance. This juice will neutralise and alkalise the body as it contains alfalfa sprouts and apricot kernels. All sprouts – alfalfa, sunflower, pea, broccoli, buckwheat – alkalise pH levels. I use black dinosaur kale, but if you can't source it, curly kale will do nicely. Black dinosaur kale has long, dark green leaves and can be sourced in all major supermarkets. Root ginger has numerous health benefits, too. This juice is a wonderful way to boost immunity, as you are drinking the blood of the plants.

WHAT YOU NEED

— *Handful kale*
— *2 handfuls alfalfa sprouts*
— *1 cucumber*
— *2 celery stalks*
— *5 apricot kernels (optional)*
— *Ginger, to taste*

WHAT YOU DO

1 Process the kale and sprouts through the juicer.
2 Then add apricot kernels, celery, cucumber and ginger.
3 Return the pulp to the juicer to squeeze out more juice.

Root ginger will not only fire up the digestive juices, it also has aphrodisiac properties.

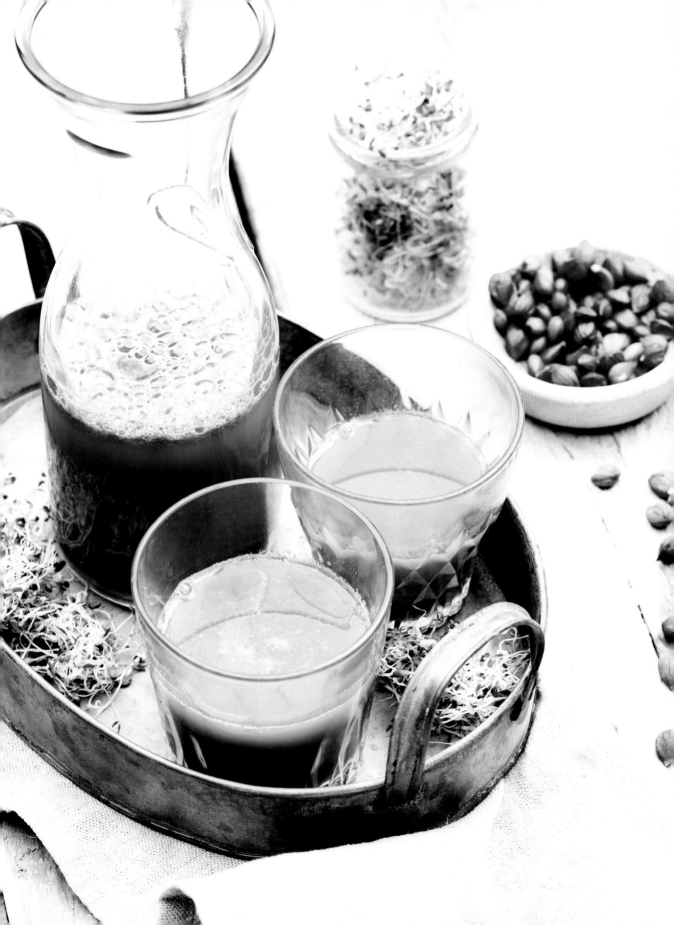

SIMPLY APPLE & LEMON

HEALTH ENHANCER

Although they say 'an apple a day keeps the doctor away', apple juice has a very high sugar content. While fructose is natural, it will spike blood sugars. Always dilute fruit juices with water to reduce this problem. I use the seeds of the apples in the juice, as they contain nitrilosides that are powerful in fighting disease.

WHAT YOU NEED

— *2 apples*
— *½ lemon, with skin*

This juice is simplicity itself, and the ingredients are readily available, but do try your best to buy organic. Be observant and wary of chemically sprayed fruits. If you cannot source organic fruit and veggies, then peel them. I know you lose a lot of nutrients when you peel fruits, but if they are sprayed it cannot be removed by washing.

WHAT YOU DO

1 Wash all the ingredients and process them through the juicer. Simple!

CLEANSE & HEAL JUICE

IMMUNE BOOSTER

I use this juice every day as it ticks both boxes. It is wonderful for cleaning out the digestive tract and healing the system. This is the main juice used at the Hippocrates Health Institute, as it is packed with chlorophyll. An increasing volume of research shows that consuming foods that are rich in chlorophyll neutralises free-radical damage in the body. Oxygen-free radicals attack many parts of the body and contribute to heart disease and cancer, and speeds the ageing process, especially in the joints. Try lemon or lime to vary the taste.

WHAT YOU DO

1 Process all ingredients through the juicer.
2 If the cucumber is large enough, this recipe will serve 2 people.

WHAT YOU NEED

— 1 cucumber
— 2 celery stalks
— Handful sunflower sprouts
— ½ lemon, with skin

Cleanse and heal at the same time with just two green juices each day.

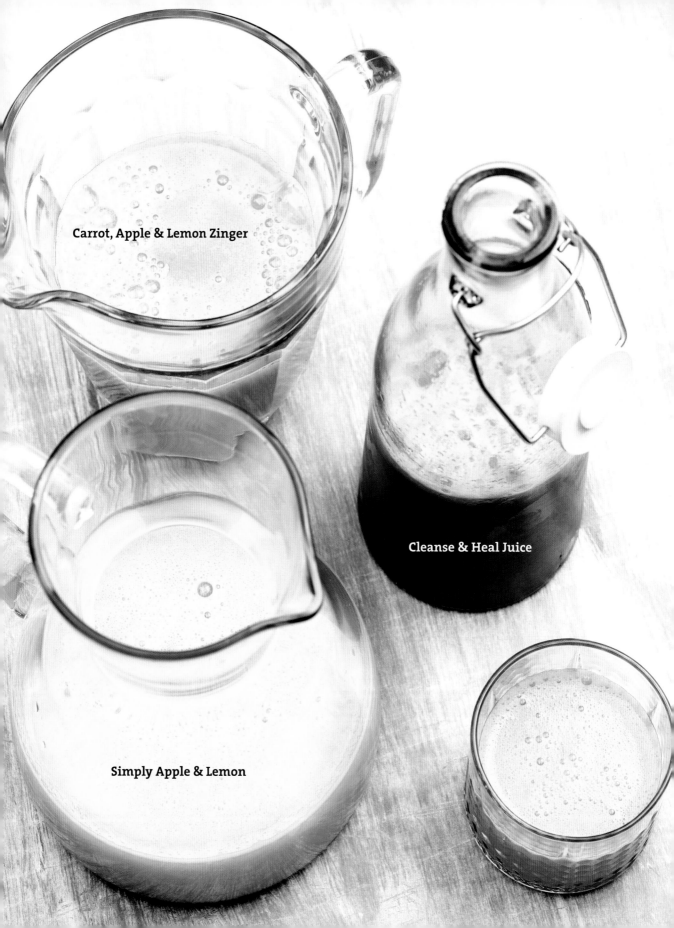

Carrot, Apple & Lemon Zinger

Cleanse & Heal Juice

Simply Apple & Lemon

CARROT, APPLE & LEMON ZINGER

HEALTH ENHANCER

If you are just starting to juice, you can mix small amounts of fruits in with the veggies. The sweet fruits will encourage a good juicing regime and, as you progress, you can gradually phase out the fruits in favour of vegetables. Add some water to dilute the sugar content of the juice.

This juice is good for your bones as it's rich in absorbable calcium, unlike many synthetic supplements, which are secreted by the body because they cannot be absorbed. I use half a lemon to give the juice a nice tangy taste.

WHAT YOU DO

1 Simply wash the ingredients, process them through the juicer and top up with water.

WHAT YOU NEED

— 2 carrots
— 1 apple (including seeds)
— ½ lemon, with skin
— 60 ml water

A lovely, colourful juice that appeals to kids, and you can be sure that it will help them to build strong bones.

YUMMY MUMMY JUICE

IMMUNE BOOSTER

If you are a busy mum trying to keep up but still want to get 'the glow', try this quick and simple juice. I know how mornings can get crazy busy, and there can be no time to take care of yourself. This juice is the healthiest fast food for people who are constantly on the go, so make a big jug and dish it out to the whole family. You can even take it with you in the car if you are short on time. Use an airtight lid to limit oxidation, and add some ice to keep it as fresh as possible.

Celery is rich in calcium, iron, magnesium, potassium and zinc; these minerals are the building blocks of cells, bones, hair, skin, teeth, nails, brain function and sexual health. Lettuces contain silica, which is great for connective tissue and a clearer complexion. The mint adds a lovely fresh flavour to this juice.

WHAT YOU DO

1   Process all ingredients through the juicer. *Voilà!* You're done and out the door.

WHAT YOU NEED

— *1 cucumber*
— *3 celery stalks*
— *Handful lettuce*
— *Handful mint*

Shop healthily if you want to look your best, and make sure your shopping basket includes lots of fresh veggies. These foods will inject vitality into your life, and soon you will be glowing all over.

NATURE'S TONIC

In wheatgrass, Mother Nature has given us one of the most nutrient-dense, vitamin-packed plants – and no, it does not taste like lawnmower clippings.

Wheatgrass juice is a real pick-me-up, especially if you are feeling run-down, sluggish or lethargic. Phytochemical analysis has revealed the presence of flavonoids, alkaloids, tannins, saponins and sterols in fresh wheatgrass juice. These compounds boost immunity and feed your cells.

It is a bit of an acquired taste, so if you are not used to wheatgrass juice, add some lemon or ginger for extra flavour. Some people feel nauseous after drinking even a small shot of wheatgrass juice; this is because of the detoxifying effect it has on the body. To eliminate this problem, try adding a little water to dilute the juice – and hang in there, it will soon pass.

WHAT YOU NEED

— *1 shot of wheatgrass (about ⅓ of a tray)*
— *¼-inch piece of ginger or a squeeze of lemon*
— *Crushed ice (optional)*

WHAT YOU DO

1   Cut and wash the wheatgrass and put the spiky end through the juicer.
2   Add the ginger and process.
3   Pour over some crushed ice, if you like.

You can grow your own, (see p. 47) or buy online. For details, see the Resources section.

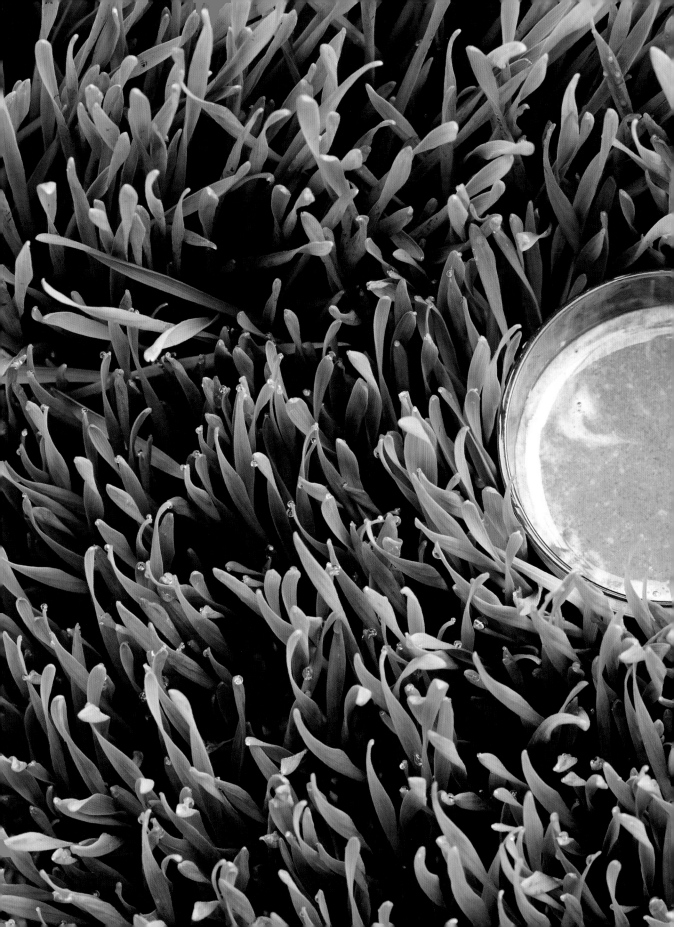

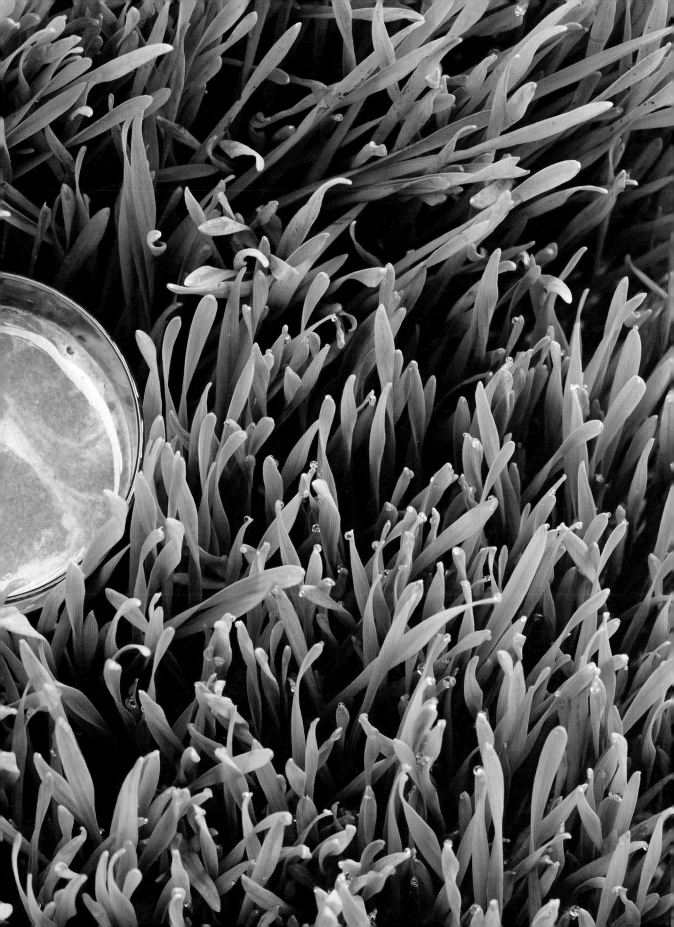

SWEET & REFRESHING MOJITO

HEALTH ENHANCER

Although this drink has no alcohol, as would a traditional mojito, be assured you will find it just as refreshing. You can whisk up this 'mocktail' of mint, stevia, zesty lime and cooling sparkling water in minutes. I played with the quantities to perfect this virgin mojito, so if you want to raise a glass but don't want the alcohol, or are abstaining for health reasons, you won't feel left out with this fabulous drink.

WHAT YOU NEED

— *250 ml lime juice*
— *500 ml sparkling water*
— *10 drops stevia*
— *handful mint leaves*
— *2 handfuls crushed ice*

WHAT YOU DO

1 Blend the lime juice, stevia and sparkling water together. Crush the mint leaves.
2 Pour the mix over crushed ice in 2 cocktail glasses. Stir everything together and serve.

A 'mocktail' is a nice treat for party guests who prefer not to drink alcohol or who are driving. Grab a straw and raise a glass!

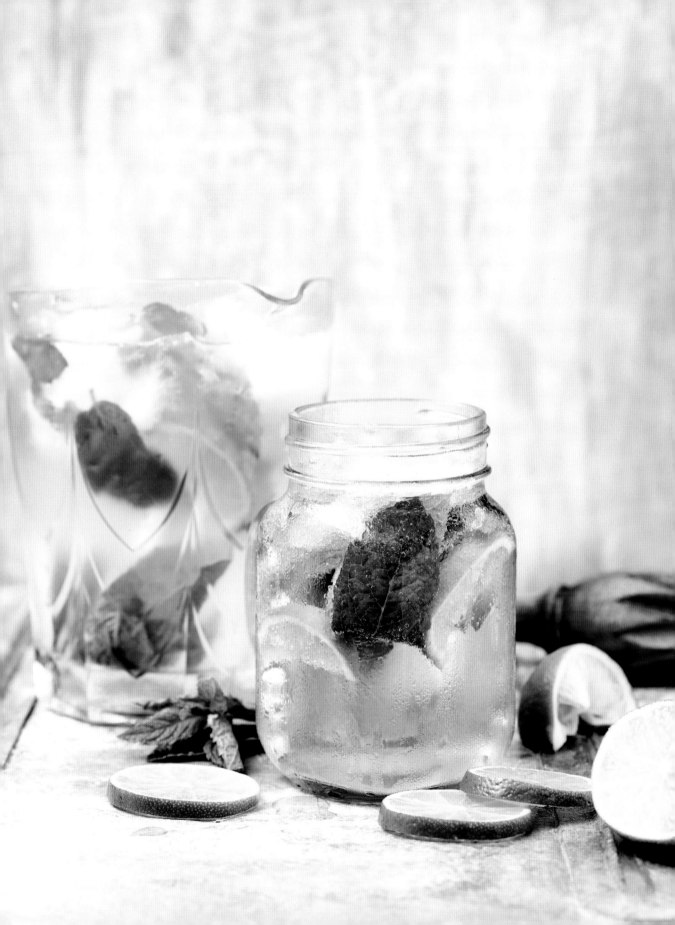

BLISSFUL VIRGIN MOCKTAIL

HEALTH ENHANCER

The tart taste of the grapefruit blended with the sweet strawberries in this drink is blissful. You can still enjoy a cocktail while looking after your health and waistline. I find I no longer get 'funny looks' and 'odd comments' for not drinking alcohol. Nowadays people are much more accepting when you say no to alcohol. Whatever your tipple, this fabulous drink is sure to please and, if you are not a drinker but want to join in the party scene, give this a shot.

WHAT YOU NEED

— *200 g strawberries*
— *1 grapefruit, peeled*
— *250 ml sparkling water*
— *Dash lime juice*
— *Handful crushed ice*

Remember, this refreshing drink is a treat, so don't overdo it just because its sweetness comes from natural sugars.

WHAT YOU DO

1 Juice the strawberries and grapefruit.
2 Add the sparking water and lime.
3 Pour over crushed ice.

SUGAR-FREE LEMONADE

IMMUNE BOOSTER

Nothing tastes the same as homemade lemonade – it's a refreshing thirst-quencher on a hot summer's day. My girls love it and start each day with a glass of freshly squeezed lemon with a dash of stevia. Lemons are great for your skin, as they cleanse and detoxify the body. The vitamin C content of lemons not only helps to stave off colds, it is also very effective in helping us to metabolise calcium. Drinking more water is a step in the right direction that is guaranteed to boost health and immunity. If you find it difficult to drink water, add some stevia to sweeten it – that should do the trick.

WHAT YOU DO

1 Juice enough unpeeled lemons to produce 250 ml juice.
2 Add the juice, liquid stevia and water to a jug to the desired strength. If the lemonade is not sweet enough for your taste, add a little more stevia to the mix.
3 Add ice cubes and lemon slices and serve.

WHAT YOU NEED

— *250 ml lemon juice, including skins*
— *1 litre cold water*
— *5 drops liquid stevia*
— *2 handfuls ice cubes*
— *Lemon slices (to serve)*

Use the skins of lemons as well, as they are loaded with phytonutrients.

SOOTHING TEAS

Teas can have a very calming and soothing effect on the body. They can soothe a sore throat or cold, calm the digestive system, alleviate constipation and give you a nice pick-me-up. It's easy to make your own tea from simple ingredients such as lemon, ginger, mint, cinnamon, cloves or turmeric. Chop your favourite ingredients, throw them all into a tea pot of hot water for a few minutes, and then strain the flavoured water into your favourite cup. These freshly made teas are naturally caffeine-free and have a lovely aroma. There is nothing I like more than to sit back and relax with a nice cuppa; here are my favourites.

WHAT YOU NEED & WHAT YOU DO

Lemon & ginger

As you know, lemon is a rich source of vitamin C and is also alkalizing. Ginger is wonderful for digestion: just one cup of this tea can settle stomach aches, pains, cramps or heartburn. It can also help soothe colds, sore throats and inflammation. Grate a small piece of ginger and squeeze ½ a lemon into a mug, and top with warm water.

Fresh mint

Mint is great for relieving headaches and reducing the symptoms of a fever or flu, as it's rich in potassium, calcium and vitamin B. Mint has a high menthol content, which refreshes the breath and aids sleep. It's so easy to grow mint in a pot on your window-sill, too. Pick a few leaves and throw into a pot of hot water and wait a few minutes – simple.

Raspberry leaf & cloves

This tea is said to help throughout labour and increase the flow of the mother's milk. The leaf is readily available in health stores. Throw a teaspoon of the leaf in a pot and add a few cloves. I remember my mother gave cloves to me as a child to relieve a toothache and ease the pain. These herbal remedies were passed on through generations. I wonder if she knew that cloves were antimicrobial, antiviral, antifungal and anti-inflammatory.

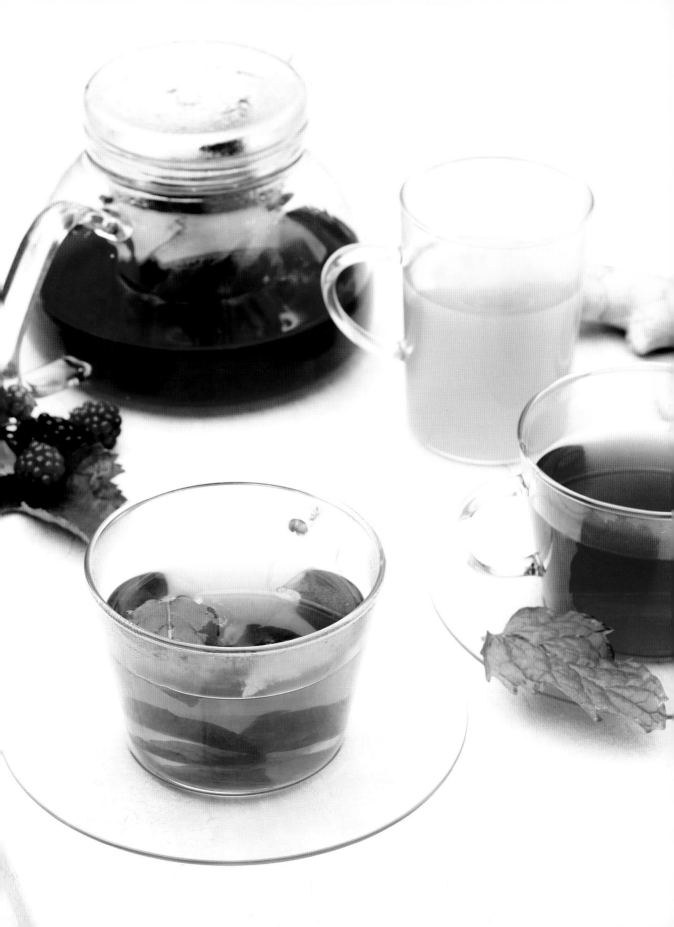

THE
LOWDOWN ON
WHEATGRASS

Wheatgrass juice is packed full of enzymes, oxygen, phytonutrients, proteins, vitamins and minerals such as calcium, magnesium, phosphorus, potassium, zinc and selenium. It's a major source of chlorophyll, which is highly effective at eliminating stored toxins and purifying the liver. It's also a valuable source of vitamin B-17, a substance that is thought to destroy cancer cells. In fact, recent studies have shown that wheatgrass is so powerful that 28 ml of it is said to be the equivalent of about 2.5 kg of fresh fruit and vegetables in terms of vitamin, mineral, trace elements and phytonutrients, which all help to increase vitality and cell health.

Basically, the wheat grains are grown in seed trays using organic compost for about ten days. When you add moisture to make the seeds germinate, their dormant enzymes spring to life and produce a huge amount of life force. It's much better to grow your own or buy online as the grass is more potent when it is juiced fresh and drunk straight away. People often buy powders and wheatgrass tablets thinking it's the same as freshly squeezed juice, but a lot of nutrients are lost in the pasteurisation and drying process of wheatgrass products.

The juice is derived from squeezing fresh wheatgrass through a masticating juicer. When it comes to juicing grass, the juicer is very important, because the cheaper centrifugal juicers cannot extract juice from the strong grassy fibres. The fibres just get stuck and can jam the machine. A masticating juicer, on the other hand, grinds the grass slowly and extracts the juice without destroying the precious nutrients. Masticating juicers also give a much better yield of juice – a shot of juice is about 30 ml and, roughly speaking, one tray of wheatgrass yields approximately three shots from a masticating juicer.

Some people like to drink it neat. I find the taste too sweet for my liking, so I mix it with lemon or ginger. Ginger root is an excellent anti-inflammatory. I absolutely love adding it to my green veggie juice, too. It gives it a lovely warm taste, especially in the winter months when drinking cold juices can seem unappealing. Ginger is also very effective in treating morning sickness, as it blocks a neurotransmitter that can trigger nausea. I well remember how my mother used to give me a warm ginger drink for a queasy stomach. She seemed to instinctively know what foods help specific ailments – there was no Google back when I was a kid.

Follow the tips below to keep the growing process simple. That way you're more likely to continue growing your own.

Wheatgrass does not contain gluten, so if you are gluten intolerant you don't have to worry.

WHAT YOU DO

1 Soak the wheat berries in water overnight in glass jars with mesh lids.
2 The jars should be placed at a 45-degree angle so the water drains off fully.
3 Rinse and drain the wheat berries daily.
4 After a day or two, small shoots will appear.
5 Fill a tray ¾ full with soil and mist it heavily with water.
6 Spread the soaked berries evenly over the soil and press gently.
7 Cover with an empty tray and place it in the dark for two days.
8 Mist the seeds with water once a day.
9 After about two days, the wheatgrass should begin to appear.
10 You can then place the tray in indirect sunlight.
11 Continue growing for a further six days, watering once daily until the grass reaches approximately 18 to 25 cm in height.
12 The wheatgrass is now ready to be used for juicing.
13 Cut the wheatgrass off with a sharp knife close to the soil and gradually feed the grass into the juicer.

WHAT YOU NEED

— *180 g winter wheat berries*
— *sprouting jars (see p. 17)*
— *35 cm seed tray (available from garden centres)*
— *A small bag of organic soil (available from garden centres)*
— *Spray bottle with water (for misting the seeds)*

You can let the tray continue to grow, as you will get a second cutting from each tray.

Bottoms up!

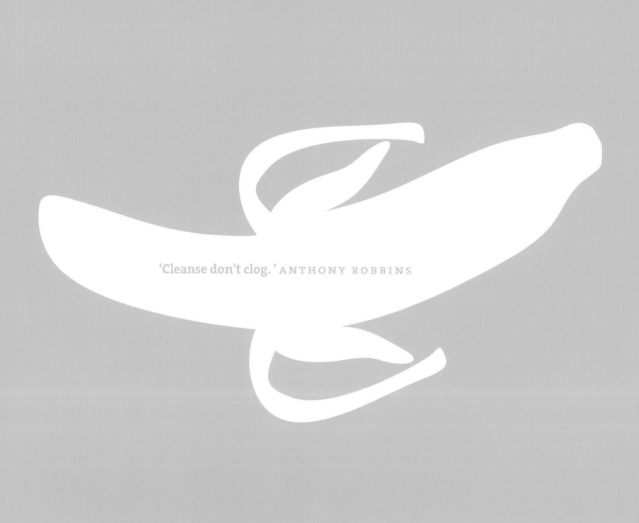

'Cleanse don't clog.' ANTHONY ROBBINS

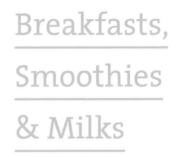

Breakfasts, Smoothies & Milks

They say that breakfast is the most important meal of the day, but I am not sure I would agree with that. You may think that I am not in my right mind, challenging the idea that breakfast is an important meal. I know it goes against the long-held theory that skipping breakfast means you tend to eat more food than usual at lunch, or gorge yourself on scones and bikkies on your coffee break, but I have my reasons.

Firstly, skipping breakfast is not as bad as you think, when you consider that most people grab a piece of toast gulped down with a mug of coffee – not much nourishment in that. Then we have the highly processed, sugar-loaded cereals that are fortified with synthetic nutrients – not much nourishment in them either. My main reason for skipping the 'normal' breakfasts is that our body cleans the colon between 11 pm and 11 am, so when we eat breakfast, we slow down the cleansing and eliminating process.

Dr Kellogg, the famous surgeon and the creator of Kellogg's Corn Flakes, believed the colon was the origin of most diseases, and he had a point, as most of the toxins in the colon come from the foods we eat. Cleansing from the inside is every bit as important as showering or brushing your teeth.

Start your day with two glasses of water and lemon juice. Drinking water is a great way to hydrate and cleanse your body first thing in the morning. Lemons also help the cleansing process. This is such a simple tip but nonetheless an important one. Drinking water early in the day helps your body kick start the cleansing and elimination process. Water is essential for eliminating waste substances and toxins from the colon.

Green juices made with cucumber help to clean out the intestines and remove waste from the colon. Juices and smoothies are great for breakfast as they have a high water content and are easy to digest. If you want to wake up your taste buds, a nice, dairy-free, frothy smoothie will start the day well. It can be difficult to change our views about dairy because we have been taught throughout our whole lives that milk is a healthy food. You can use rice, oat or almond milks. These milks can be bought in all the main supermarkets or health stores, or you could make your own if you are pressed for time. Nut milks are packed with protein and can be used for smoothies or poured over cereals.

Try the Moo-free Shake, it's great if you are vegan or lactose intolerant. My daughter Sarah uses almonds as they have a nice flavour and creamy texture. Add some stevia to give it a hint of sweetness, or vanilla extract and cinnamon; they make a really nice combination and are a good alternative to sugar. Cinnamon has many medicinal uses and helps with colds, nausea, diarrhoea and painful menstrual cramps. Raw bee pollen is also wonderful for sweetening smoothies and cereals.

Even if your mornings are frantic and crazy busy, green juice is the healthiest fast food for those who are constantly on the go. Kids can have juices and smoothies to fuel their growing bodies and developing brains, and they can drink it in a handy cup on their way to school if you are short on time. Chia seeds are a healthy addition to shakes, and are a great way to add good fats to your diet; they are rich in anti-oxidants and a good source of omega-3. Soak the chia seeds overnight, so they can be added to smoothies or porridge. Alternatively, the ground seeds can be sprinkled on cereals. Udo's oil can also be used in smoothies – it is a rich source of good fats, and is wonderful for your skin and hair.

Organic strawberries and raspberries are at their best when they are in season. However, they are not always available, so make the most of them when they are in season because they are amazing for your skin. They help promote the production of collagen, which is a part of the connective tissue that helps the elasticity and constant renewal of skin cells. Raspberries clear out nasal passages of mucus.

Most people assume that they will pay hugely inflated prices for organic foods, but even if you are on a tight budget, you can eat organic foods. I am often asked if it's worth spending extra money on organic produce, and my answer is always YES. Consider the long-term dangers of pesticides: neurological symptoms, immune system disorders, liver disease and asthma attacks. Can we honestly believe that there is no threat to our health if our bodies' resources are spent trying to get rid of chemicals from food?

Something else I really enjoy in the morning is cherry tomatoes. Tomatoes are a fruit, so they should always be eaten on an empty stomach. They are a rich source of vitamin C and lycopene, which helps to mop up damaging free radicals in the body that can harm our cells. They are low in calories and fat free. Talk about fast food for breakfast – a quick rinse under the tap and they're ready.

If you are unwavering in your belief that breakfast is the most important meal of the day, try the Powerful Quinoa Porridge – it is a big hit with my youngest daughter. Don't be afraid to try new grains like millet, buckwheat, teff and quinoa if you prefer a cereal-based breakfast. These grains will give you sustainable energy to get you through the morning. Unlike many store-bought cereals on the market, there are no hidden sugars or synthetic nutrients. These grains are a nourishing, wholesome and satisfying way to start out your day.

LEAN & GREEN SMOOTHIE

IMMUNE BOOSTER

This plant-powered green drink is great for those who find it difficult to get enough greens into their diet. My lean and green smoothie is alkalizing, cleansing and loaded with phytonutrients, antioxidants, and essential vitamins and minerals. The best thing about this smoothie is it's fruit-free. The addition of coconut milk is fantastic for hydration, building lean muscle and helping to keep those hunger pangs away.

WHAT YOU DO

1 Chop the cucumber and blend with the spinach and coconut milk until smooth.
2 Next, pit and peel the avocado and add to blender.
3 Squeeze in lemon juice and blend again.

WHAT YOU NEED

— ½ cucumber, chopped
— 450 g fresh spinach
— 250 ml tinned coconut milk
— ½ avocado, pitted and peeled
— ½ lemon

You can buy coconut milk in most supermarkets these days.

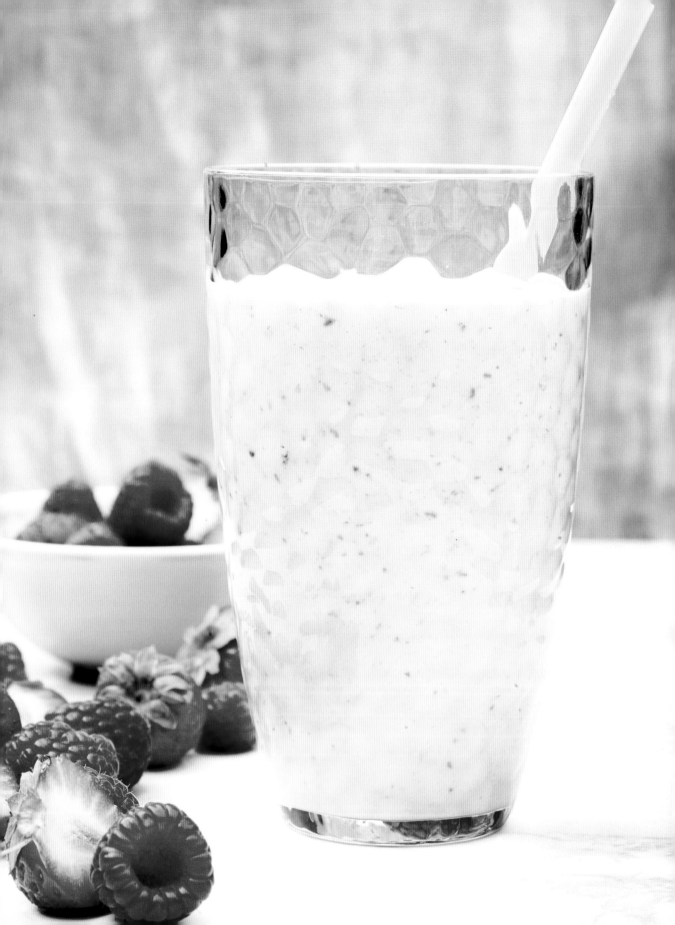

MOO-FREE SHAKE

Sometimes I have to get creative to keep my youngest daughter Julie interested in preparing her own healthy foods. As I tried to nurture her passion for healthy foods, we came up with this berry smoothie. She has moved on now to green drinks, but this one helped her through the transition phase. If you are lactose intolerant, this smoothie is made with moo-free ingredients. Berries are amazing for your skin as they help promote the production of collagen, which is a part of the connective tissue that helps the elasticity and constant renewal of skin cells.

WHAT YOU DO

1 Bend all the ingredients until the desired consistency is reached.
2 Add ice and serve.

WHAT YOU NEED

— *50 g strawberries*
— *30 g raspberries*
— *60 ml water*
— *1 banana*
— *3 drops stevia*
— *Handful ice*

Fussy, picky eaters will love this smoothie.

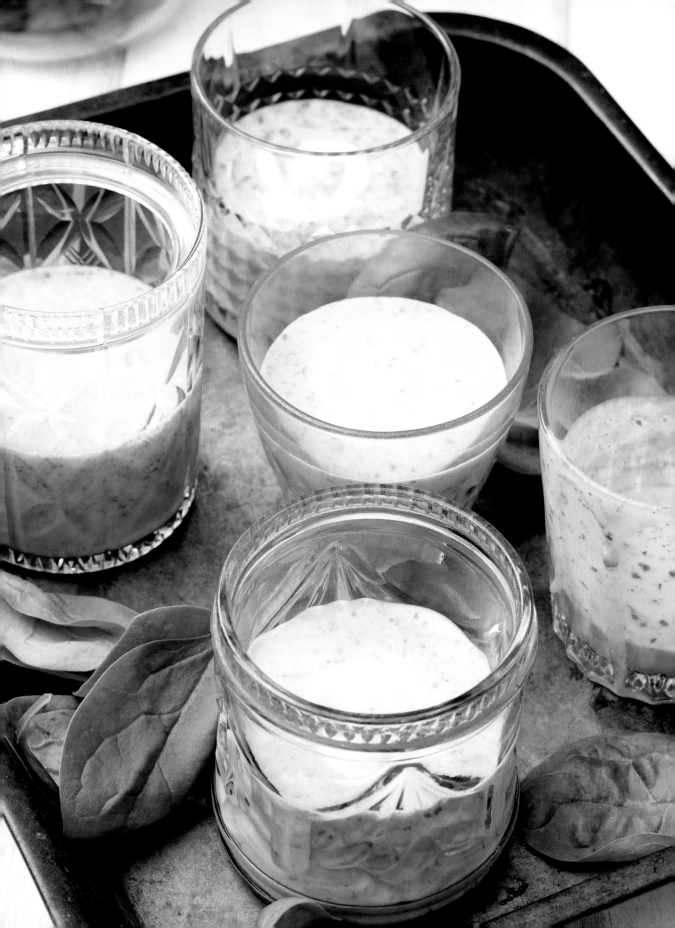

GET UP & GO SHAKE

HEALTH ENHANCER

Who would think that spinach would work well in a smoothie? I came up with this dairy-free shake in an effort to move my children away from store-bought yoghurts that contain so much sugar. Most commercial yoghurts contain as much as 30 per cent sugar. You will have no problem encouraging kids to take good bacteria and essential fats for breakfast with this yummy drink. Whisk it up in no time – in fact, it's faster than either cereal or toast to put together. Good bacteria are a healthy addition to shakes, and are a great way to add good fats to your diet. Udo's oil can be used in smoothies – it is a rich source of good fats and is wonderful for your skin and hair.

WHAT YOU DO

1 Blend all ingredients together until smooth.
2 Pour over some ice and you're ready to go.

WHAT YOU NEED

— *1 banana*
— *125 ml coconut milk*
— *Small handful spinach leaves*
— *1 tsp Udo's oil or ½ tsp chia seeds (soaked)*
— *Ice, to serve*

A lack of essential fats can lead to cravings, as the body needs a regular supply of good fats from foods in order to thrive.

RESVERATROL-RICH SHAKE

Resveratrol is a phytonutrient found in the skin of red grapes that is associated with positive health effects. It acts as an antioxidant and anti-inflammatory, and may reduce the risk of heart disease and cancer.

However, there is a catch: grapes are high in natural sugars, so enjoy this delicious shake in moderation. Coconut milk is an ideal choice for dairy- or soy-sensitive people; it is rich in calcium, iron, magnesium, potassium, phosphorus, zinc, manganese, copper and selenium. Blend well to make sure there are no chunks of skin in the smoothie from the grapes.

WHAT YOU NEED

— *100 g red grapes*
— *125 ml coconut milk*
— *½ tsp Udo's oil*
— *Handful ice*

WHAT YOU DO

1 Blend all the ingredients until the desired consistency is reached.
2 Add a handful of ice and stir.

If you want to wake up your taste buds, this refreshing smoothie will do just that.

SUGAR & SPICE DELIGHT

IMMUNE BOOSTER

Has the mention of sugar got your attention? I use stevia to give this milk its sweet taste. Nut or grain milks are great to add to breakfast cereals for a wonderful brekkie combo. If you are lactose intolerant, this is a great alternative source of milk. I know, I know, you may say you have no time to make homemade milk, but think of the benefits! You can make a batch that will last for three days in the fridge, and it's well worth the effort.

Cinnamon has anti-bacterial, antiviral and antifungal properties.

WHAT YOU DO

1 Soak the nuts overnight in water. Rinse and strain off the water and discard.
2 Blend all the ingredients in a blender until roughly mixed.
3 Strain through a fine-mesh sieve, nut-milk bag or muslin.
4 Retain the nut pulp, as it can be added to cookies or pâté. The milk will last for two or three days when refrigerated.
5 Add stevia to taste, and sprinkle with cinnamon (optional).

WHAT YOU NEED

— 140 g pre-soaked almonds
— 500–750 ml water
— 3 drops stevia
— Cinnamon (optional)

This milk has a lovely flavour and creamy texture. The cinnamon and stevia give it a hint of sugar and spice.

DAIRY-FREE YOGHURT

IMMUNE BOOSTER

I like to add bee pollen to this yoghurt for kids, as it sweetens it and adds colour. Kids love colourful food, and this one is loaded with nutrients. At first, I thought making your own yoghurt would be laborious, but I wanted to find a way to make sugar-free, non-dairy yoghurt because there is so much sugar in the store-bought varieties, and sugar encourages the growth of harmful bacteria. The coconut milk is easily sourced in supermarkets.

WHAT YOU NEED

— 125 ml coconut milk
— 1 handful pine nuts
— ½ tsp vanilla extract
— ½ tsp Udo's oil
— 1 tsp raw bee pollen (optional)

Add some Udo's oil to the mix to ensure you get a daily dose of essential fatty acids.

WHAT YOU DO

1 Place all the ingredients into a blender and blend until you get the consistency of creamy yoghurt.
2 Add a little extra coconut milk until you get the desired consistency.
3 Pour over your favourite breakfast cereal or enjoy on its own.

ENERGY-BOOST GRANOLA

HEALTH ENHANCER

Even if you have only a few minutes to eat breakfast, at least make it one that's good for you. This energy-boosting granola will give you a very satisfying start to your day. It is rich in zinc magnesium and vitamin E, and a powerful antioxidant with anti-cancer properties. It is loaded with enzymes, as the seeds are sprouted, and is free of gluten, dairy and refined sugar.

WHAT YOU DO

1 Soak the seeds and buckwheat overnight and rinse the following morning.
2 Leave to drain while you prepare the fruit.
3 Mix the seeds and fruit together and drizzle rice milk on top.
4 Pour over some delicious dairy-free yoghurt, and serve!

WHAT YOU NEED

— *100 g buckwheat, soaked overnight and rinsed*
— *140 g sunflower seeds, soaked overnight and rinsed*
— *150 g pumpkin seeds, soaked overnight and rinsed*
— *4 dates, chopped*
— *2 tbsp blueberries, washed*
— *rice milk, to serve*

You can dry the buckwheat in the dehydrator if you prefer a crunchier breakfast.

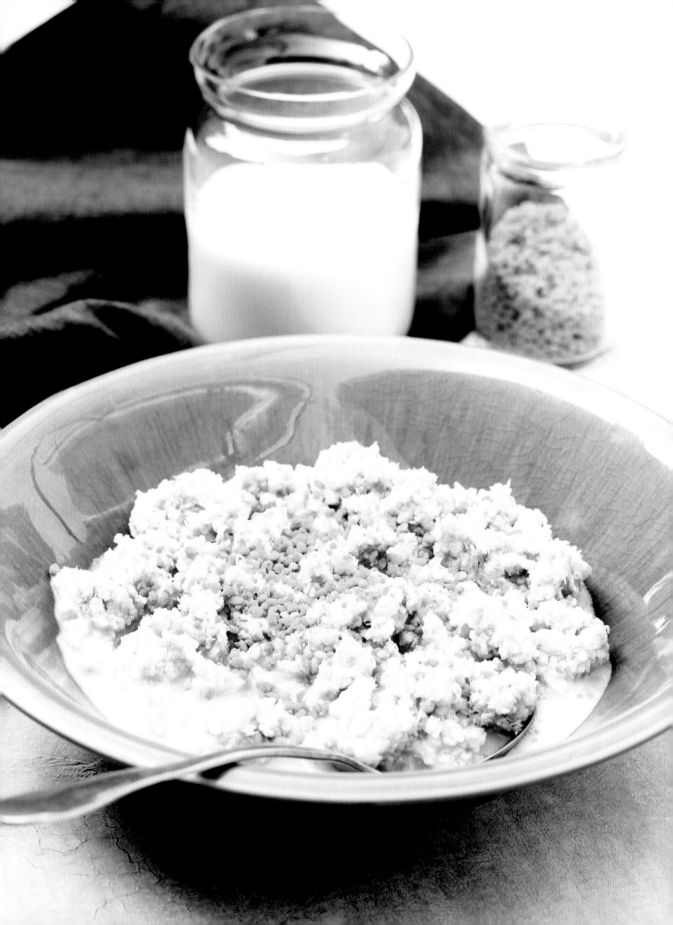

FULL-OF-FIBRE PORRIDGE

IMMUNE BOOSTER

If you like a cereal-based breakfast, millet is a super grain to add to your diet. It's a nourishing, wholesome and satisfying way to start out your day, and a good filler for hungry tummies. Millet is rich in fibre, which studies show offers significant protection against breast cancer for pre-menopausal women. Soluble fibre has been shown to lower cholesterol and protect the heart.

I always soak seeds and nuts overnight, but millet gets smelly if soaked for long periods, so rinse it well and only make enough for two days.

WHAT YOU DO

1 Soak the millet overnight, drain the water and rinse thoroughly.
2 Warm the millet with some water in a small pot till it forms a nice, soft, creamy porridge.
3 Drizzle some stevia or nut milk over the top, if desired, and sprinkle with bee pollen.
4 Spoon into a bowl and serve.

WHAT YOU NEED

— *425 g millet, soaked and rinsed*
— *3 drops stevia*
— *2 tsp bee pollen*

Don't be afraid to try new grains; they really have outstanding nutritional benefits.

POWERFUL QUINOA PORRIDGE

IMMUNE BOOSTER

As chillier temperatures set in, many people like a warm breakfast to set them on their way. Quinoa is a powerful source of protein; in fact it's a complete protein, which means that it contains the nine essential amino acids that the body needs to repair itself. Quinoa is gluten-free and a good source of fibre, which sweeps the gut of unwanted waste. It's also much more digestible than the normal oat porridge.

WHAT YOU NEED

— *80 g flaked quinoa*
— *250 ml water*
— *Sprinkle pumpkin seeds*
— *2 or 3 drops stevia (optional)*

The stevia adds a lovely natural sweetness, so you don't need to add sugar – you know, the totally addictive stuff.

WHAT YOU DO

1 Warm the quinoa flakes and water in a small pot till it forms a nice, soft, creamy porridge.
2 Drizzle a few drops of stevia over the top, if desired, and sprinkle with pumpkin seeds.
3 Spoon into a bowl and serve.

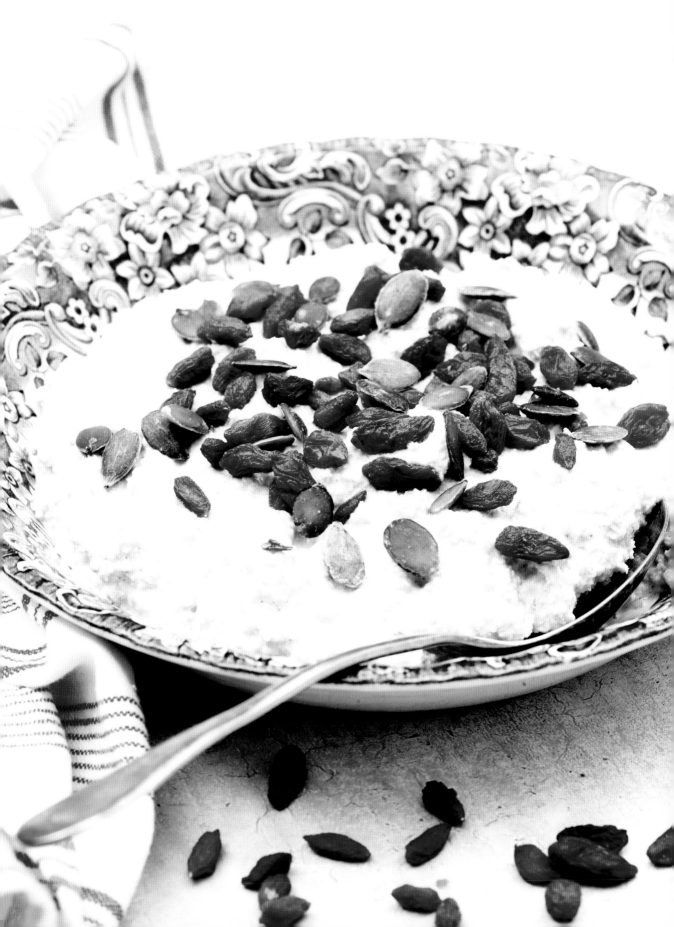

WHEAT-FREE BREAKFAST

IMMUNE BOOSTER

Buckwheat lowers blood sugars more slowly than wheat-based cereals. With a low glycaemic index, it may be helpful in the management of diabetes. It also improves appetite, is great for digestion and good for drawing out excess fluid from swollen areas of the body. Buckwheat is loaded with an impressive array of useful minerals such as calcium, iron, magnesium, potassium, zinc, copper and manganese, in addition to proteins and antioxidants. I like to add some dairy-free yoghurt to this dish; its natural, sweet flavour will start out your day on the right foot. You can make several batches at a time and store in a glass container.

WHAT YOU NEED

— *250 g buckwheat*
— *250 ml almond milk*
— *dairy-free yoghurt, to taste*

Contrary to what its name suggests, buckwheat is not wheat; it's actually related to rhubarb. It's gluten-free and great for those who are gluten sensitive.

WHAT YOU DO

1 Soak the buckwheat in water for an hour.
2 Rinse off the starchy soaking water.
3 Drain and place the buckwheat on parchment paper on a dehydrator tray.
4 Dry overnight till crunchy.
5 Drizzle the dairy-free yoghurt over the crunchy buckwheat, and serve with almond milk.

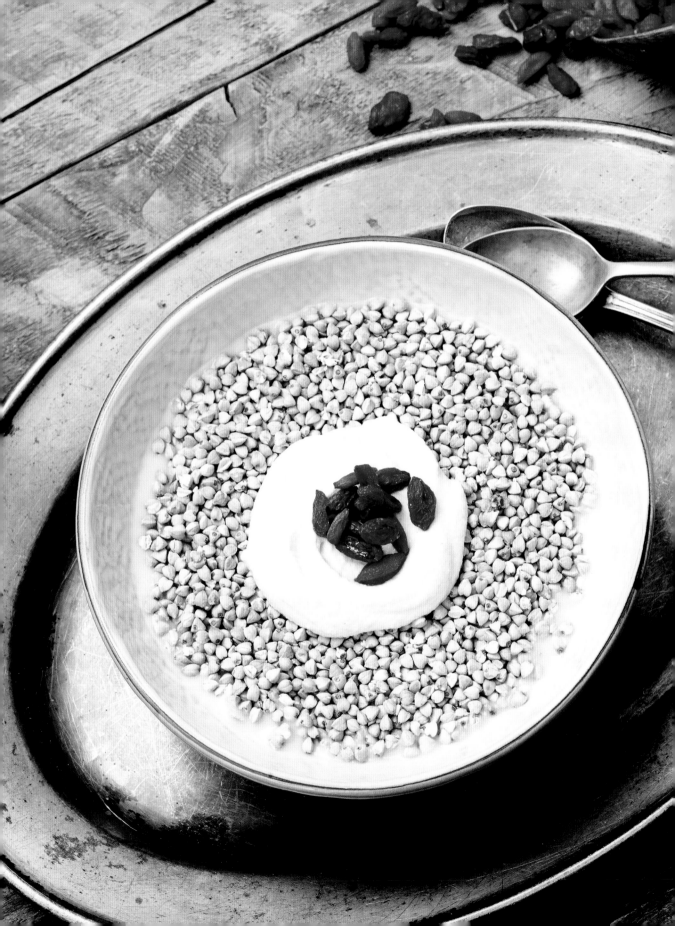

'My weaknesses have
always been food and
men – in that order.'
DOLLY PARTON

Hot &
Cold Soups &
Appetizers

Winter brings a change in weather, and we can become more susceptible to colds and flu. A warm bowl of soup is the traditional cure for winter chills and a great way to nourish, nurture and protect ourselves during those months. I have to say there is something about a nice warm soup on a cold winter's evening that nothing else can replicate. Bolster yourself against the chill with these delicious soups.

Cayenne pepper is fantastic for seasoning and warming up soups. It also adds a nice kick to bland meals. It's extremely spicy, so use it very sparingly until you get used to its peppery taste. I use it on nearly everything instead of pepper. Try it in hummus, soups, curries, crackers and sauces to give them extra flavour. I don't know how I ever ate food without it. It can be added to a glass of water first thing in the morning to improve circulation and help to clean and maintain the cardiovascular system. It has a variety of other therapeutic properties that has earned it its healing reputation, including calming ulcers, lowering blood pressure, and it is used to coagulate blood in cuts and wounds.

In this section you will find both cooked and raw soups, which will help to ease you in gently to eating raw. The reasons people follow a raw diet vary from weight loss, health benefits, energy levels, to its anti-ageing properties. Eating raw can make a big difference for those who are trying to lose weight or who want to drop a size – this I discovered quite by accident when I changed my eating habits. It is a delicious, easy way to boost your health and lose weight without bingeing and dieting.

Adding more veggies to your meals also reduces the amount of carbs on your plate. We assimilate carbs better from plants, sprouted grains, pulses and vegetables, and they have a low glycaemic load. If you restrict your carbohydrate intake to what you burn daily, you will not gain weight. Bread, pasta, potatoes, biscuits and crackers are all major sources of carbs. The good news is that dieting becomes a thing of the past when you move to raw foods, and you will soon enjoy floods of compliments coming your way as people notice your new slim figure, glowing complexion and superb energy levels.

Good fats are also important for weight loss; they keep us slim, help with weight management and they can also improve a sluggish metabolism. Good fats noticeably increase metabolic rate and energy levels, which, in turn, help us to burn more calories. Most people don't really understand the difference between good fats and bad fats. Even the word 'fat' makes us assume that fats make us fat, but that is not always the case. Naturally, if you think fats are going to make you fat you will try to avoid them, but fats do not make you fat, excessive carbohydrates make you fat.

The misunderstanding about the differences between good fats and bad fats has led to the majority of the population trying to avoid all fats, but good fats are necessary for good health. They increase our energy production by helping the body to obtain more oxygen, and when we have increased energy levels, we feel much more active. This, in turn, means that we are less likely to crave sugar or carbohydrates to deal with energy dips.

Removing good fats from your diet can, in fact, make it difficult for your body to lose weight. Ironically, if we avoid good fats, we get fatter, because we need fat to burn off excess fat. We must remember that small amounts of fats are an intrinsic part of a healthy body – it is not only our figures that suffer from abstaining from these foods but also our health. Good fats are also beneficial at keeping your hair shiny, your nails strong and your skin young-looking and blemish-free.

One of the best strategies you can employ if you feel you are overweight is to add more raw foods into your diet. Raw veggie soups are truly nutritious, because raw soups retain the enzymes and nutrients that are otherwise lost when they are cooked. They are also filling and taste great. It is so easy to add real, nourishing foods into your day-to-day routine, but you need to ensure that you are enjoying it, as well as benefitting from it. Food needs to be tasty! I tried these recipes out on my teenage daughter, Julie, and she loves them. I use coconut milk, squash, seaweeds, spices and herbs to add flavour to these easy recipes. Try the Super Seaweed Soup – it's fantastically nutritious, tasty and, as an added bonus, it's very quick and easy to prepare.

If you prefer something warm, you can always opt for the cooked soups. I know that when you live in a cold climate, the thought of salads and raw foods may not be appealing. Winter weather makes us crave comforting, hot dishes. This is where a dehydrator comes in very handy. Dehydrating warms the food and helps to transform veggies into a 'meal'. When warmed, the veggies look and taste like cooked foods. Eating foods prepared in this way starts the process of eating for health rather than comfort, because you are eating foods without destroying their valuable nutrients.

If you are on a tight budget and you want to add a filling, nourishing soup to your menu, the Nurturing Pea Green Soup is both cheap and cheerful. If you are worried that your family will turn up their noses, I guarantee this delicious soup will be a major hit.

Here are three tips for eating more raw, living foods throughout the chillier weather:

- Add more chilli, cayenne pepper and ginger to your foods.
- Warm plates and bowls before serving.
- Put warm sauces over your salad.

SUPER SEAWEED SOUP

IMMUNE BOOSTER

A quick, super-nutritious soup for those days when you are ravenous and need something instantly. Seaweeds offer great protection against radiation so, if you travel by air, sit in front of a computer or have had radiation treatments, they are worth adding to your diet. The coconut gives some metabolic-boosting medium chain triglycerides. I like to alternate between dulse, kelp and nori seaweeds to get the minerals and trace minerals that are often lacking from our diet.

WHAT YOU DO

1 Soak the wakame and dulse seaweed in a bowl of tepid water for about 15 minutes while you peel the ginger and chop the avocado.

2 Drain the water from the seaweed and remove any excess water with a kitchen towel.

3 Blend the seaweed, coconut, avocado, ginger and lemon juice together until you get the desired consistency.

4 Add paprika and stevia, if desired, to taste, and serve immediately.

WHAT YOU NEED

— 10 g dulse seaweed
— 10 g wakame seaweed
— 1 avocado, peeled and destoned
— 200 ml coconut milk
— 1 tsp ginger, peeled and finely chopped
— ½ lemon, juiced
— 3 drops stevia (optional)
— Pinch paprika (optional)

For those of you who have never tried seaweed soup, this might be the time to give it a go.

NURTURING PEA GREEN SOUP

IMMUNE BOOSTER

I have included this recipe because it is a huge family favourite in the winter months, and I had such feedback from my readers who just loved it. It's nurturing, filling and really cheap to make. With just three very cheap ingredients – peas, onions and vegetable stock – this soup is great value for money. I serve this to friends and family on cold evenings or for a satisfying lunchtime filler.

WHAT YOU NEED

— *450 g dried green split peas*
— *2 onions*
— *1 tbsp vegetable bouillon powder*
— *1.25 litres boiling water*

Dust with paprika or cayenne pepper before serving to give the soup a warm effect and colourful appeal.

WHAT YOU DO

1 Soak the dried peas in cold water for about an hour to soften them. Drain off the soaking water.

2 Melt the stock in the boiling water and pour over the peas. Peel the onions, cut into slices and add to the peas and stock.

3 Bring to a gentle simmer. Cover and cook for a further 20 minutes until all the peas and onions are tender.

4 Blend the soup until smooth, adding more stock if the soup is too thick.

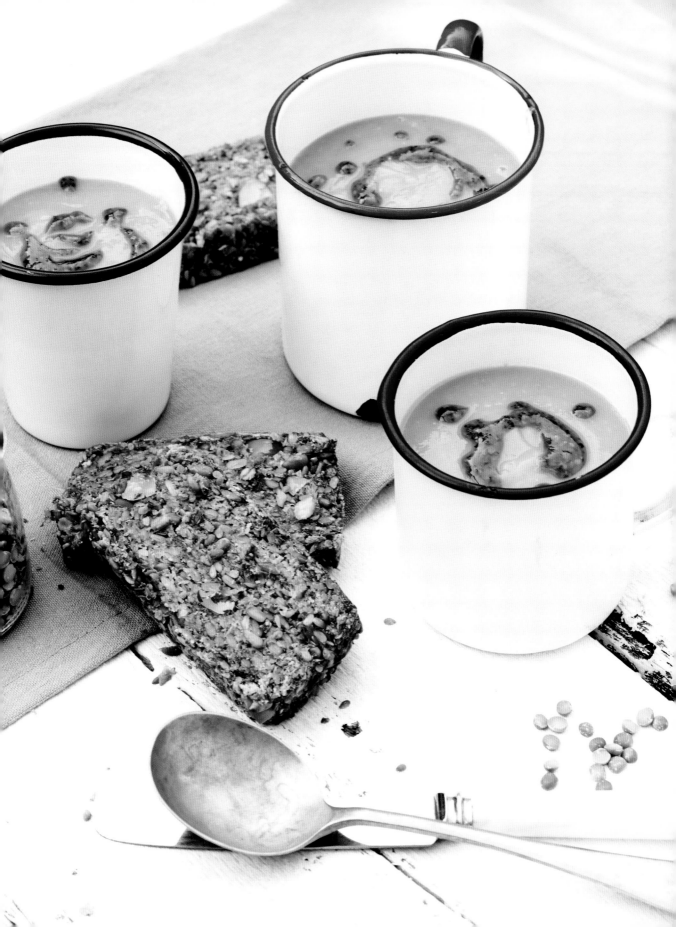

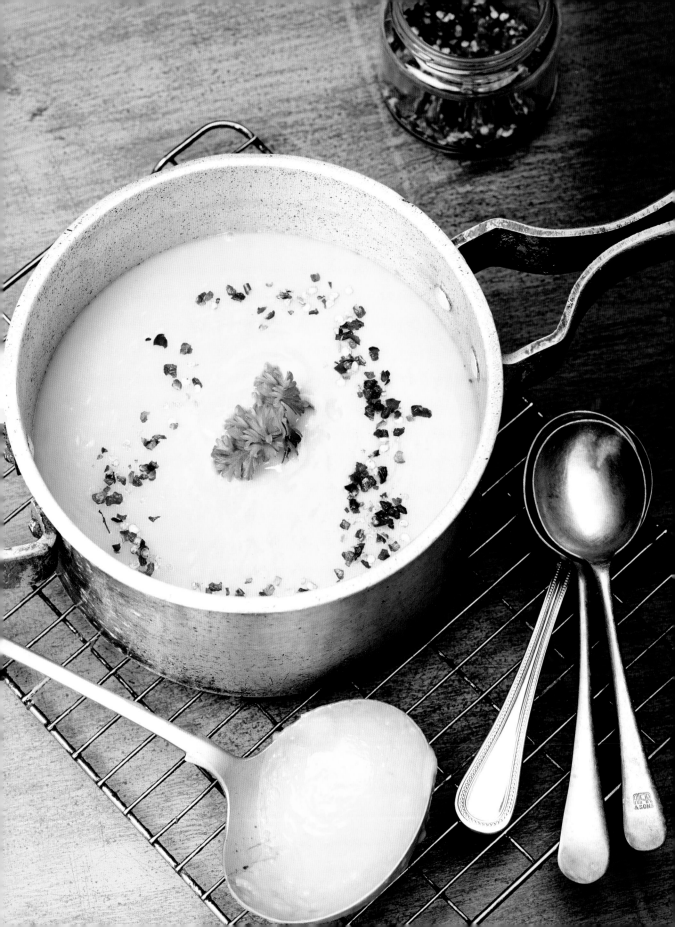

POSH SOUP

IMMUNE BOOSTER

This soup is posh enough to serve at dinner parties or special gatherings. It was an instant hit with my friends and family, and I am sure you will absolutely adore it. Sweet, rich and creamy, you would almost think it was made with full-fat cream. I prefer to use water instead of oil to cook the onions, because oils heated to high temperatures form harmful by-products.

To make this soup a little fancier for special occasions, drizzle a little of the coconut milk on top and garnish with a few chopped chilli flakes.

WHAT YOU DO

1 Remove the skin and seeds from the squash and peel the onions.

2 Cut the onions and squash into slices. Cook the onions gently for a few minutes in a small amount of water, stirring regularly to prevent the vegetables sticking.

3 Melt the bouillon powder in the boiling water and pour over the onions. Add the chopped squash and coconut milk and bring to a gentle simmer.

4 Cover and cook for a further 20 minutes until all the vegetables are tender.

5 Blend the soup until smooth, adding more stock if the soup is too thick.

6 Add chilli flakes before serving.

WHAT YOU NEED

— 1 butternut squash
— 400 ml tin coconut milk
— 2 onions
— 1 tbsp vegetable bouillon powder
— 250 ml boiling water
— Chilli flakes, to garnish

This soup needs to be a part of your posh food repertoire. It will definitely earn you praise.

SWEETCORN CHOWDER

IMMUNE BOOSTER

This raw soup is fantastically nutritious and tasty, and, as an added bonus, it's very quick and easy to prepare. It's wonderful if you have an unexpected visitor for lunch and have to improvise with store cupboard ingredients. The idea behind this soup I owe fully to Renate, a talented chef at the Hippocrates Health Institute. I first ate this soup in Renate's home; her inspiring dishes are awesome.

Avocados are staples among raw-food enthusiasts. The avocado and corn is a great combination of flavours, and the almond milk combines equally well.

WHAT YOU NEED

— 240 g sweetcorn
— 500 ml almond milk
— ½ avocado
— 250 ml water
— 2 spring onions
— Pinch turmeric
— Pinch garlic powder
— Pinch cayenne pepper

Raw soups are such a tasty change from the over-cooked soups that have become the norm.

WHAT YOU DO

1 Peel and destone the avocado, and wash the spring onions.
2 Put all the ingredients in a blender and blend until smooth.
3 Add a little warm water if the soup is too thick.
4 To add extra colour to this rich and creamy soup, sprinkle with spring onions or cayenne pepper to serve.

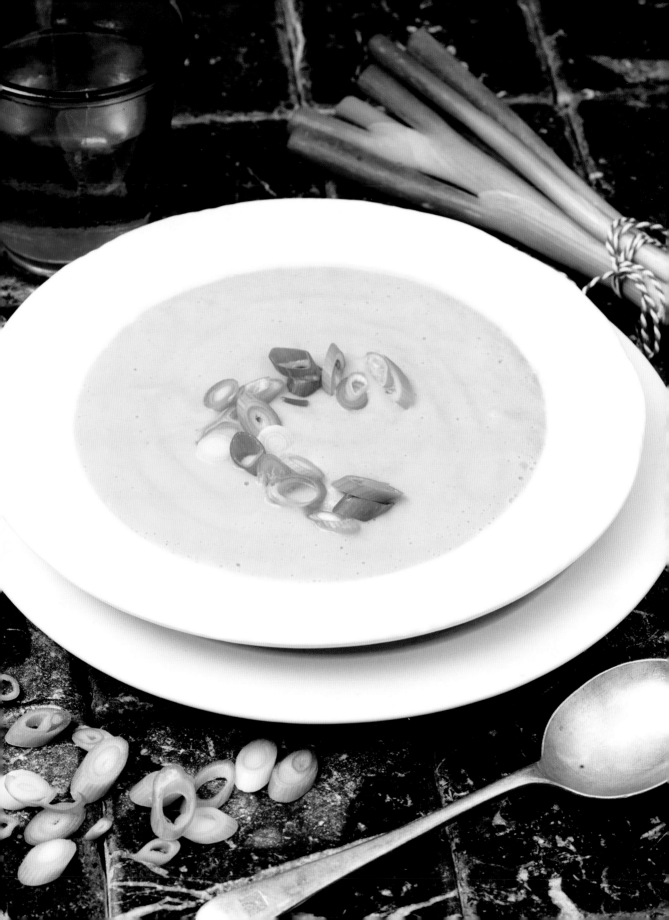

BETA-CAROTENE SOUP

IMMUNE BOOSTER

Carrots rank high on the list of antioxidant vegetables in this truly nutritious soup, and beta-carotene helps to reduce the risk of cardiovascular disease. It's the avocado that gives this soup its creamy texture; they're rich in omega-3 fatty acids and vitamin E, which is great for your skin and hair.

If you prefer a warm soup, add some warm water to this recipe.

WHAT YOU NEED

— 1 avocado
— 2 small carrots
— 200 ml coconut milk
— 1 tsp ginger, finely chopped
— ¼ lemon
— 3 drops stevia (optional)
— Pinch paprika

WHAT YOU DO

1 Peel the avocado, carrots and ginger. Remove the stone from the avocado.
2 Put all the ingredients in a blender and blend until smooth.
3 Add a little warm water if the soup is too thick.
4 Sprinkle with paprika to serve.

Raw soups are so easy to prepare, you simply throw everything into a blender and whizz. Sooooo easy.

DELICIOUS MELON GAZPACHO

IMMUNE BOOSTER

Melons are rich in potassium, beta-carotene, lycopene and vitamin C; these nutrients may control blood pressure, regulate your heartbeat and reduce the risk of prostate, breast and endometrial cancers.

If you are used to fasting throughout the week, this melon gazpacho is a great way to break a fast as it replenishes electrolytes and tastes delicious. I add stevia and a pinch of celery salt to balance the flavours.

WHAT YOU DO

1   Peel and de-seed the melon.

2   Chop into chunks and blend.

3   If the gazpacho is too thick add a small amount of water.

4   Add stevia and celery salt to taste, and serve garnished with some fresh mint.

WHAT YOU NEED

— *1 medium cantaloupe melon*
— *A little water, for blending*
— *Few drops of stevia*
— *Pinch celery salt*
— *Fresh mint, to garnish*

Cantaloupes continue to ripen when picked from the vine, but ripe melon should be eaten as soon as possible. You will love this gazpacho, it's delish.

VITAMIN D STUFFED MUSHROOMS

IMMUNE BOOSTER

Mushrooms are rich in vitamin D; they have figured out how to get vitamin D from the sun even though they grow in the shade. Vitamin D helps us to absorb calcium, so it's important to include it in our diets. Some mushrooms have very high levels of vitamin D, like morels, chanterelles and shiitake, though they can be very pricey, so use the best, freshest mushrooms you can.

The stuffing is very substantial, and you can also use it to fill courgettes. It's a great stuffing if you are trying to eliminate bread.

WHAT YOU NEED

— 12 mushrooms, cleaned
— 60 ml Bragg Liquid Aminos
— 60 ml olive oil

WHAT YOU NEED FOR STUFFING

— 70 g pine nuts
— 1 red pepper
— 1 tsp Udo's oil
— Fresh herbs: basil, oregano, sage

WHAT YOU DO

1 Clean the mushrooms and marinate in Bragg Liquid Aminos and oil for 20 minutes, tossing gently from time to time.

2 Process the nuts, herbs and red pepper, adding the oil last.

3 Stuff each mushroom with about half a teaspoon of the mixture.

4 Place in dehydrator for 1 hour.

Serve this with a sprouted salad for a truly delicious and satisfying filler.

POTASSIUM-RICH CELERY 'SALT'

IMMUNE BOOSTER

'Each year, food companies use an amount of salt that is every bit as staggering as it sounds: 5 billion pounds.' – Michael Moss

Why not try making your own (salt-free) celery salt? It really is simple. Why bother? Well, table salt (sodium chloride) has been linked to heart disease, muscle cramps, arthritis, diabetes and cancer. It contains bleaching agents, synthetic iodine, and, last but not least, the dreaded sugar. I know, it's hard to believe. Eating excess sodium can also be harmful to people with hypertension or high blood pressure, and it causes fluid retention. Also remember that convenience foods and ready-prepared meals are high in sugars and salts.

Celery, on the other hand, is loaded with potassium; you can vary the flavour of the salt by adding garlic or onion, or make them separately. It's a fabulous way to use up wilted celery.

WHAT YOU DO

1 Chop the celery into small chunks and place on dehydrator trays.
2 Dehydrate overnight until the celery is dry and mince in a blender. How cool is that?

WHAT YOU NEED

— *1–2 bunches celery*

If you are trying to quit salt but miss flavouring your food, why not use this healthy potassium-rich celery 'salt'?

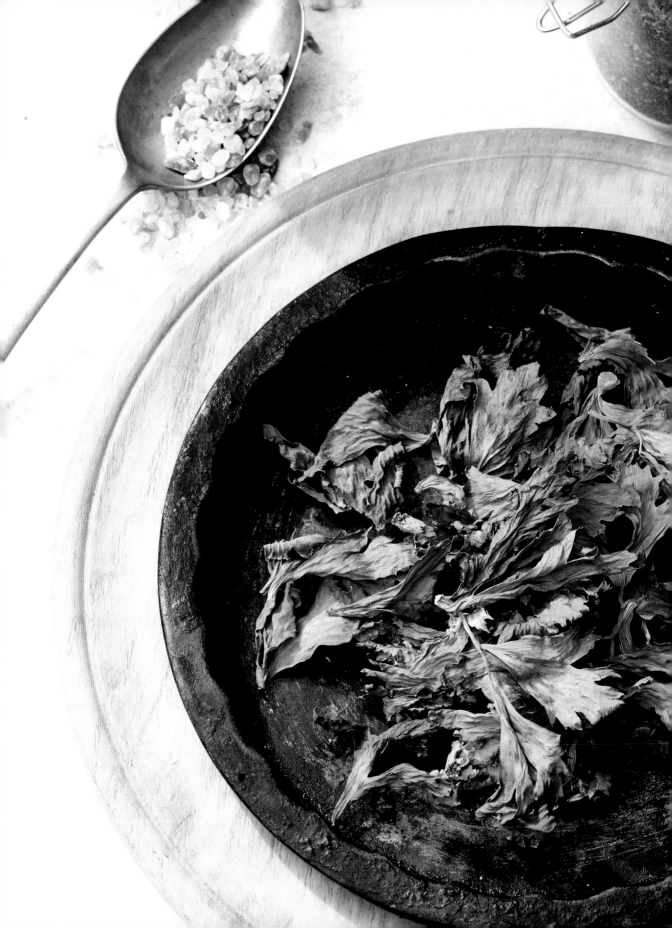

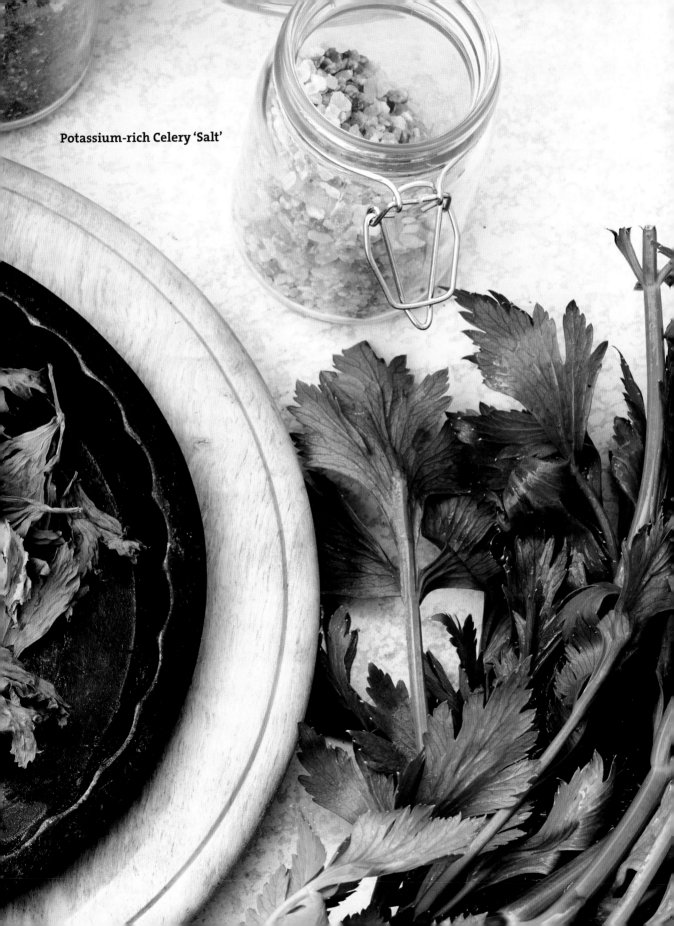

Potassium-rich Celery 'Salt'

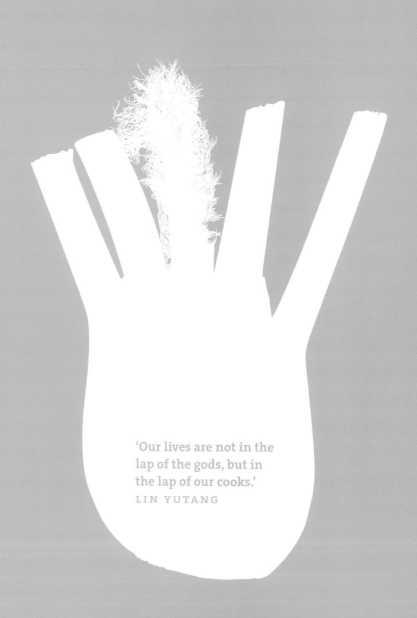

'Our lives are not in the
lap of the gods, but in
the lap of our cooks.'
LIN YUTANG

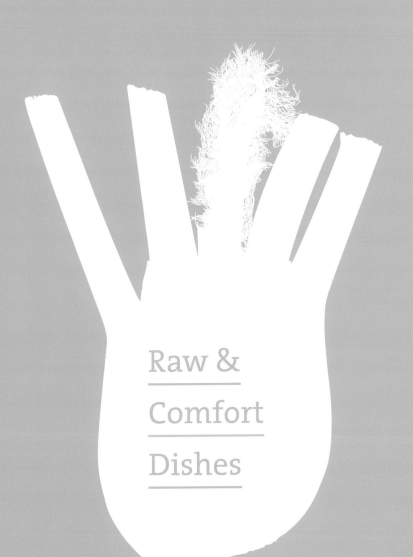

Raw &
Comfort
Dishes

Personally I find a lot of truth in this Lin Yutang quote. We need to make sure that the foods we eat are packed with enzymes, phytonutrients, vitamins, minerals and fibre that nourish us, and that usually comes down to whoever prepares our food. I have designed these recipes to include the vitamins, minerals and nutrients that we need to stay healthy.

The human body is a machine that needs the correct fuel, much like your car needs fuel, oil and water. Humans have a physiological need for enzymes, vitamins, minerals and other organic nutrients such as essential fats. These nutrients need to be supplied regularly and in high enough quantities in order to maintain a healthy body. If you deviate from the formula, you increase your chances of lowering your immune system, which is your main ally against disease.

Switching to a healthier diet consisting of at least 80 per cent raw foods naturally replenishes those vital nutrients – they offer the perfect balance. The bioavailability of nutrients in a raw diet is very high because the proteins, fats and nutrients are unaltered. It is simplicity and perfection from nature's kitchen.

Most people who make the switch live on 80 per cent raw and 20 per cent cooked. Remember, cooked foods are comfort foods, and although we may feel we need a little comfort now and then, especially when you live in a cold climate, once cooked above 40 degrees Celsius or 104 Fahrenheit, food is deficient in many vitamins, minerals, and enzymes. Even if you are eating cooked, home-made meals you cannot be sure that your nutritional needs are being sufficiently met, because the very act of cooking destroys much of what is beneficial to sustain optimum health. You should avoid microwaved foods; they might be convenient, but microwaves denature food. You may be eating foods you enjoy, but the vitamins, minerals and proteins will be destroyed.

As we humans are not carnivores, you won't find any meat, fish, chicken, eggs or dairy in my recipes; that's because anything that includes animal foods or animal products is not on my menu anymore. But it might be on yours. If you have been raised on meat, chicken, fish and dairy, you may think you will wither away if you don't get enough protein, when in fact too much protein is associated with a number of diseases. Too much protein can raise blood cholesterol levels, cause a decline in kidney function and increase the risk of calcium loss, which can lead to osteoporosis.

Protein has to be broken down into amino acids to be beneficial, and high-protein foods require a massive amount of energy to break down. To overcome the problem, your body must work overtime struggling to digest proteins, which in turn puts added pressure on the immune system. In addition to this, undigested meat can remain in the intestines and become putrefied, which leads to a toxic build up and often chronic ailments of the joints and heart set in. While chicken is not as dense as beef or pork, it has its own problems. A lot of people eat lighter meats like chicken because they believe they are a healthier option. What they don't realise is that chicken can also raise LDL levels of 'bad' cholesterol. To be frank, there is very little in the difference. Since the horsemeat scandal, where horsemeat was used in a wide range of meat-based products, thousands of households have switched to meat substitutes, with sales increasing by as much as 20 per cent. It appears that for consumers, the word 'meat' just isn't as appealing anymore. Fast food chains like Taco Bell have dropped the word 'meat' from one of their menus and opted for 'protein' instead in an effort to boost costumer appeal.

I know it might seem difficult to get past our rigid thinking that we cannot survive without meat, but we can. Many of us have had a carnivorous diet forced upon us in order to help us obtain appropriate nutrition without knowledge of the facts. Protein deficiency diseases, such as kwashiorkor or marasmus, are very rare except in countries where people are starving. The Centre for Disease Control in the US states that protein deficiency is most common amongst people in impoverished communities of developing countries, and in the elderly who do not meet their daily calorie needs. I have not eaten meat, fish or chicken for over 15 years and my health has improved dramatically in that time – and I promise you won't be living on leaves for dinner.

'Meat-free Monday' has become quite popular. It has many benefits – it's healthier, as you eat more veggies, it's cheaper, and you can reduce your carbon footprint and save precious resources of fossil fuels and fresh water. Why don't you give it a go and join the growing number of people who are moving to plant-based diets? A meat-free meal one night per week is not so difficult. There are lots of wonderful, tasty recipes to tempt you in this section. Stick with one night for a few weeks until it becomes the norm and then introduce a second meat-free meal. Gradually adding a new dish on one or two days a week will enable your taste buds to adjust.

Even a small bit of restructuring will give you a few nights each week without meat. This will give your body a well-deserved rest from digesting animal foods. Then you can try an uncooked, meat-free meal one or two nights a week. As your family starts to see and enjoy the benefits in their energy, mood, etc., you could build on it, until the majority of their meals are nutrient-rich. Soon, you will be less likely to stick something in the microwave or send out for pizza. Small and attainable steps can have a big impact on our lives, and will ultimately mean better health and fewer trips to your doctor. If you have a pressing health challenge, opt for the raw recipes.

Trust me, you will have no problem incorporating 'healthy' food into your meals when you begin to taste how delicious this food actually is. As soon as you get a feel for it, you will eat food of a far superior quality, while also saving yourself some time and money. Jazz up a simple cottage pie with some roasted garlic, learn to make raw, carb-free pasta, or spice up your life with a wonderfully hot and spicy curry. Yay!

NO-CHEESE PARMIGIANO

IMMUNE BOOSTER

This no-cheese parmigiano is just as good, if not better than the classic calorie-loaded version. It's loaded with protein and essential fatty acids. Most raw recipes for cheese use cashew nuts, but cashews cause inflammation, which accelerates the ageing process. Now I know macadamia nuts can work out to be expensive, but it's worth giving this cheese a shot, because it's delicious crumbled over pasta, salads and soups.

WHAT YOU DO

1 Soak the nuts in water for half an hour to soften. Drain well and process the nuts in a blender.

2 Add the rest of the ingredients and process until smooth and creamy. Don't over-blend or you will end up with nut butter.

3 Spread thinly on two sheets of parchment paper.

4 Dry overnight in a dehydrator until the cheese is fully dry. Crumble over pasta, pizza, salads or soups.

WHAT YOU NEED

— 280 g macadamia nuts
— 4 tbsp nutritional yeast
— 125 ml lemon juice
— 250 ml water
— ¼ tsp garlic powder

If using nutritional yeast is new to you, don't panic! It's really not difficult. It gives the parmigiano that authentic cheesy taste.

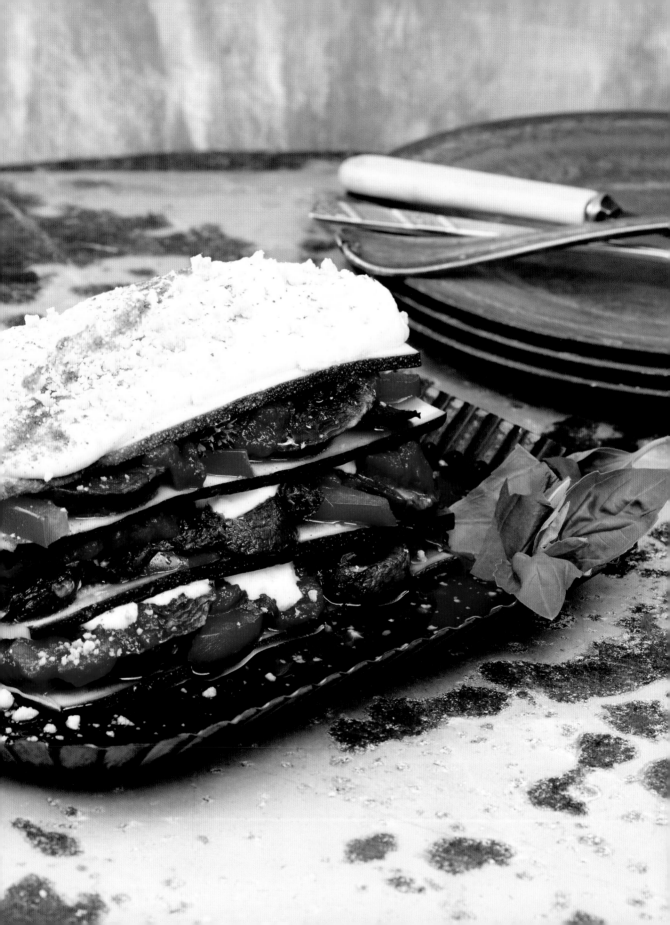

RAW-INSPIRING LASAGNE

IMMUNE BOOSTER

This lasagne is really easy to piece together, and believe me, it is awe-inspiring. There are a few different components to it, but don't let that put you off. It's a lot easier than making 'normal' lasagne, because you simply build layers of your favourite fillings. I like to use garlic mushrooms, red peppers and onions. It can be warmed in the dehydrator for 10 minutes to give it a cooked feel.

WHAT YOU DO

1 Trim of the ends of the courgettes and slice into thin strips.
2 Slice the mushrooms, onion and peppers, and marinate in garlic oil while you prepare the sauce.
3 For the sauce, process the red pepper, onion, garlic, stevia, herbs and bouillon powder together in a blender.
4 Start with a layer of courgette strips. Then add some of the marinated veggies.
5 Drizzle over the sweet pepper sauce and add another layer of courgettes.
6 Build another layer of veggies and sauce, and finish with a layer of courgettes.
7 Make the cream sauce below, and top your raw lasagne with it.

WHAT YOU DO FOR THE CREAM SAUCE

1 Soak the nuts in water for half an hour to soften. Drain well and process the nuts in a blender.
2 Add the rest of the ingredients and process until smooth and creamy.

I throw leftover pesto, spinach or basil into this lasagne to add extra nutrients. Tried and tested with my gang, who claim it to be awesome.

WHAT YOU NEED FOR THE 'PASTA' LAYERS

— *2 courgettes*

WHAT YOU NEED FOR THE FILLING

— *2 red peppers*
— *200 g mushrooms*
— *1 red onion*
— *45 ml garlic oil*

WHAT YOU NEED FOR THE SWEET PEPPER SAUCE

— *1 red pepper*
— *1 white onion*
— *2 garlic cloves*
— *1 tsp vegetable bouillon powder*
— *3 drops stevia*
— *Fresh or dried herbs: basil, oregano*

WHAT YOU NEED FOR THE CREAM SAUCE

— *280 g macadamia nuts*
— *4 tbsp nutritional yeast*
— *60 ml lemon juice*
— *250 ml water*
— *¼ tsp garlic powder*

CARB-FREE SPAGHETTI WITH SWEET PEPPER PASTA SAUCE

IMMUNE BOOSTER

Pasta doesn't have a particularly distinctive taste; it's really the sauce you use with the pasta that gives it flavour. There is no need to peel the courgettes, but if you want a white-looking pasta then peel them. Packed with veggies, this sauce works really well poured over raw courgette spaghetti. If you are not in the mood to cook, this carb-free pasta can be prepared in seconds with a simple turn of the handle. Then you can relax, as you will have no sticky pots to take care of afterwards.

WHAT YOU NEED FOR SPAGHETTI

— 2 courgettes

WHAT YOU NEED FOR SAUCE

— 1 red pepper
— 1 white onion
— 2 garlic cloves
— 1 tsp vegetable bouillon powder
— 5 drops stevia
— Fresh or dried herbs: basil, oregano

WHAT YOU DO

1 Peel and trim the ends of the courgettes and spiralise through the turning slicer with the spaghetti blade.
2 Process the red pepper, onion, garlic, stevia, herbs and bouillon powder together.
3 Gently warm the sauce, and just before serving, pour over the raw spaghetti. Kids love it!!!

I am not big on too many gadgets in the kitchen, but a spiraliser is a very handy gadget that can give you professional-looking cut vegetables and it's really easy to use. You can spiralise many different vegetables, including courgettes, sweet potatoes, carrots and butternut squash. *Voilà*!

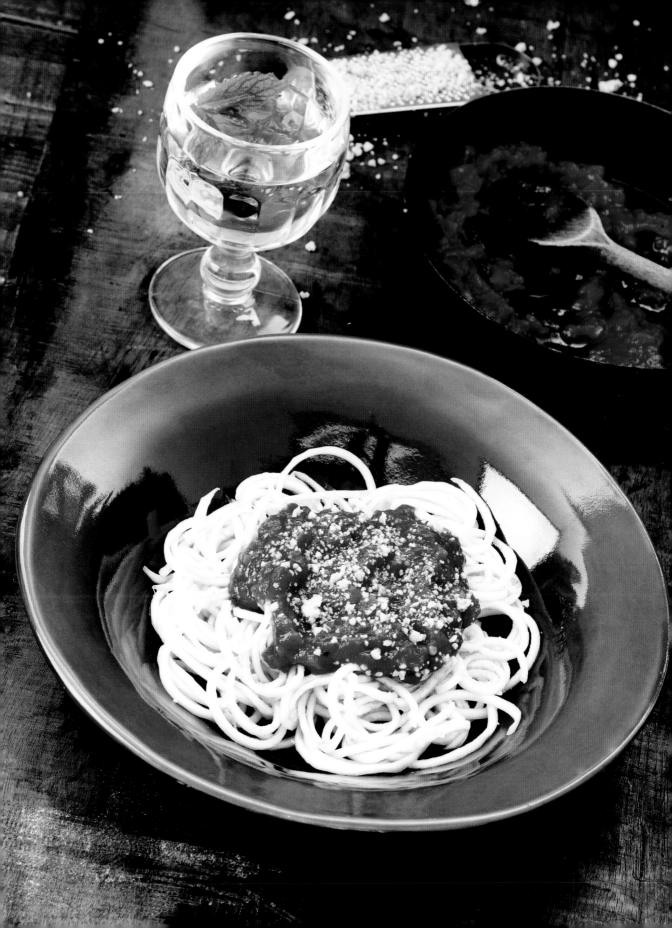

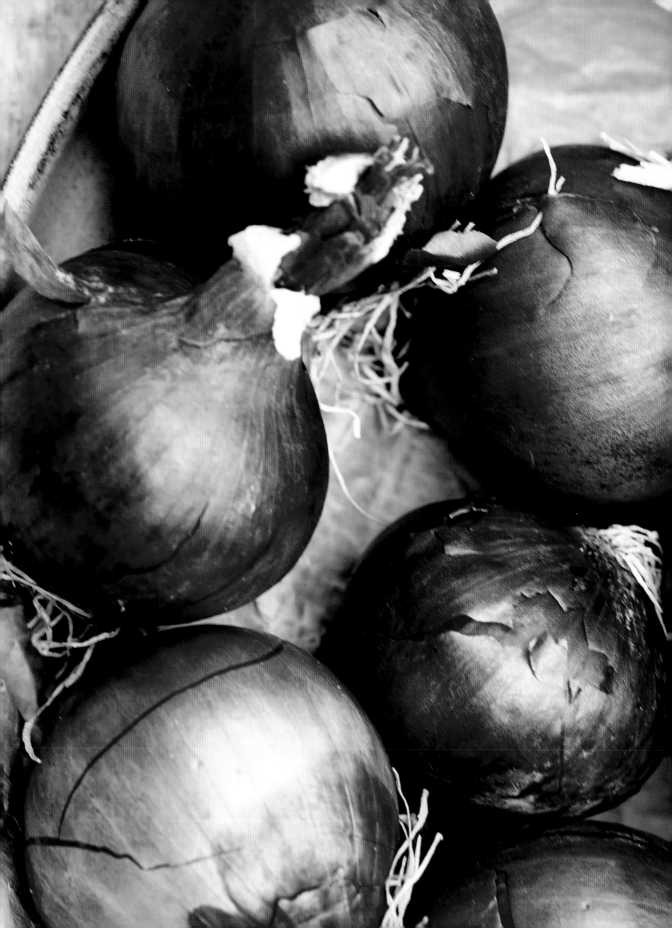

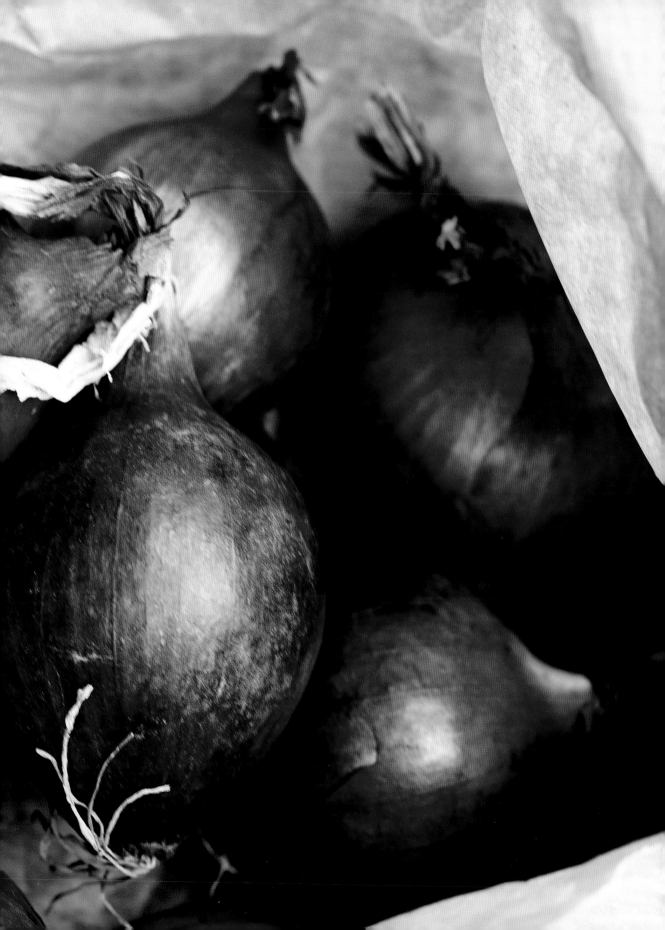

STIR, DON'T FRY

IMMUNE BOOSTER

If you love Chinese food, but want to avoid greasy take-aways, try this dish. It's not fried, so you will get all the benefits of the nutritious ingredients. It's so quick to prepare; you simply chop the veggies, mix in the oil and seasoning, and throw it on the dehydrator while you prepare some rice. It's an easy way to get your five-a-day. Remember, even if you have a hectic life, you still need to eat nourishing food.

WHAT YOU NEED

— *100 g mushrooms*
— *1 red pepper*
— *1 onion*
— *1 garlic clove*
— *250 g bean sprouts*
— *2 tbsp Bragg Liquid Aminos*
— *2 tbsp olive oil*

WHAT YOU DO

1 Chop the mushrooms, onions, garlic and red pepper into a large bowl.

2 Add the bean sprouts.

3 Coat the vegetables in Bragg Liquid Aminos and oil and place on a dehydrator tray until the vegetables become warm and slightly softened (approximately half an hour).

Quick to prepare, it will soon replace the take-away!

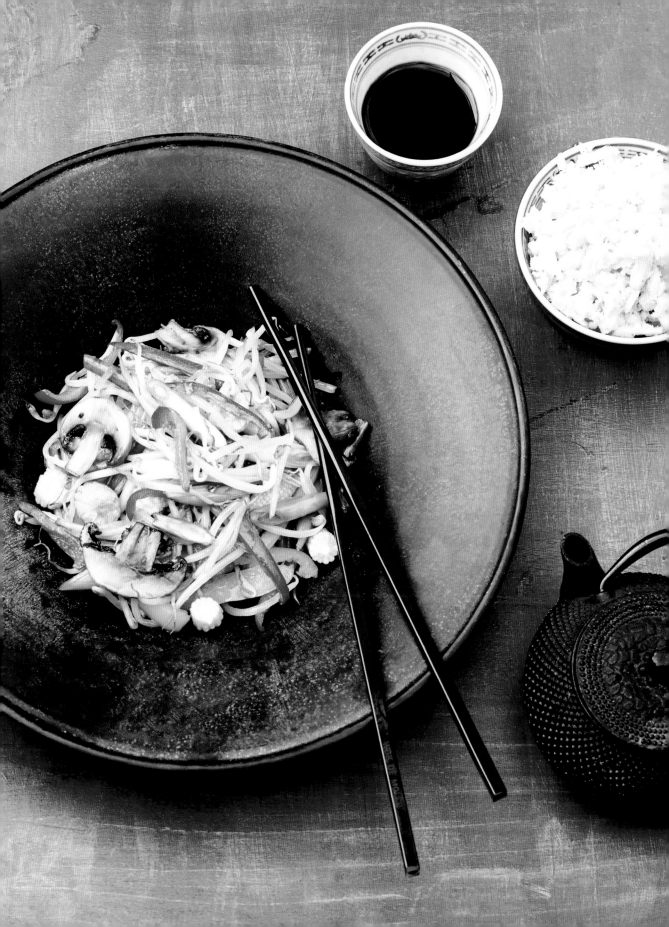

DELICIOUS TACOS

IMMUNE BOOSTER

These tacos are packed with flavour, texture and freshness. They have become a real family favourite, and they disappear in my house as soon as they hit the table. The lettuce leaves are filled with the delicious mixture and topped with strips of red pepper and a squeeze of lime. Walnuts are rich in omega-3 fatty acids. They also have higher levels of polyphenolic antioxidants than any other edible nuts.

WHAT YOU NEED

— 200 g walnuts
— 1 small onion
— 1 garlic clove, finely minced
— 2 tbsp fresh parsley
— 1 tsp Bragg Liquid Aminos
— 2 tsp chilli powder
— 6 large lettuce leaves
— 1 lime
— 1 red pepper

Serve with a scrumptious guacamole or your favourite salsa. Delicious.

WHAT YOU DO

1 Place all the ingredients, except for the lettuce leaves, red pepper and lime, in a food processor. Blend until finely chopped, but don't over-blend – leave a few chunky bits. The nuts should have a crunchy texture.

2 Place the lettuce leaves on a flat surface and add a few spoonfuls of the walnut mixture on top.

3 Chop the red pepper into strips and place over the walnut mix.

4 Add a squeeze of lime juice.

5 Roll up the leaves and serve.

BETTER THAN TUNA

IMMUNE BOOSTER

This recipe comes from a very talented chef, Renate Wallner at the Hippocrates Health Institute. It is a great example of how simple and delicious ingredients can be adapted to replace fish.

Soak the sunflower seeds the night before, rinse and drain thoroughly. With a little prep ahead of time you can then blend it together in a flash. Sunflower seeds are an excellent source of essential fatty acids; they are largely used for their edible oil on a commercial scale but are a huge source of calcium, which is so beneficial for those wanting a natural source of calcium for bone health.

WHAT YOU DO

1 Drain the sunflower seeds and process all ingredients in a blender, except celery and onions.
2 Dice celery and onions very finely to add texture to the mix.
3 Serve with salad and sprinkle with kelp powder for that authentic taste of the sea.

WHAT YOU NEED

— *425 g sunflower seeds*
— *125 ml water*
— *60 ml lemon juice*
— *1 tsp Bragg Liquid Aminos, or to taste*
— *100 g finely diced celery (optional)*
— *half a white onion, finely diced*

This dish is surprisingly filling. I love it, and I am sure you will too!

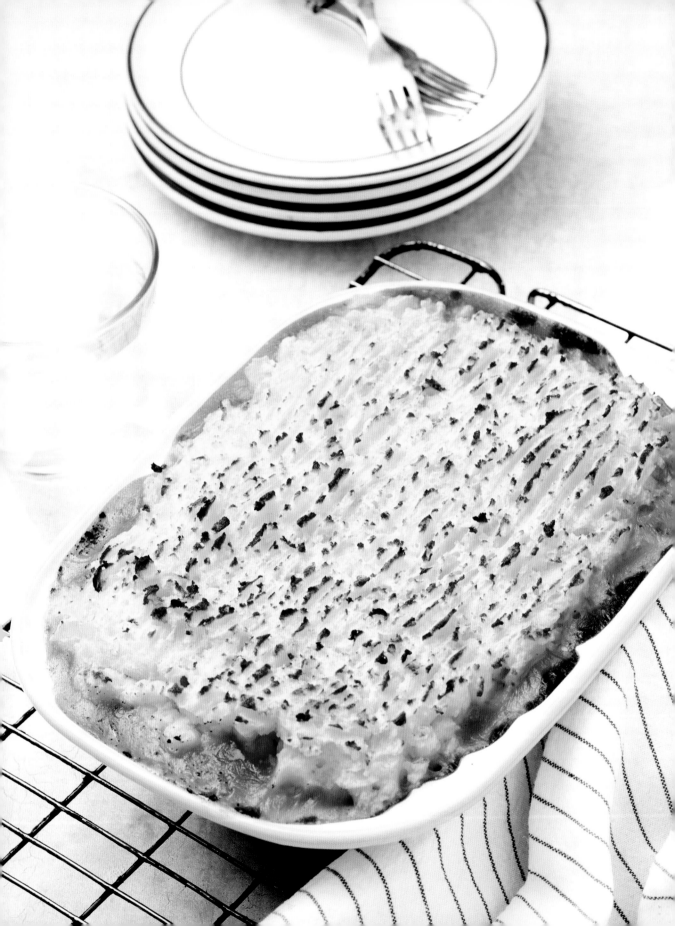

ROASTED GARLIC COTTAGE PIE

HEALTH ENHANCER

You can omit the potatoes if you are eating from the immune booster menus, but the crunchy potato topping really makes this dish. Potatoes are nightshades and contain a substance called alkaloids. Alkaloids have a negative impact on joints, nerve and muscle function. So, if you have arthritic problems, nightshades are not the best foods for you.

I use a lot of raw garlic in my salads to retain all its nutrients, but here I have roasted the garlic to give this dish a different twist. You can always vary this recipe with a different range of seasonal vegetables; it's great for using up the leftovers from your fridge.

This pie is ideal when you crave some hearty, rustic, warming food.

WHAT YOU DO

1 Roast the garlic in the oven and peel and chop the veggies into bite-sized pieces.

2 Cook the onions in a pot in a small amount of water at a medium heat for about two minutes. Stir constantly to prevent sticking.

3 Blend the vegetable bouillon powder with the water and pour over the onions.

4 Throw in the veggies and herbs and reduce the heat.

5 Blend the gram flour with a small amount of hot water and add to the vegetables to thicken the sauce. Allow the stew to simmer for 30 minutes.

6 Meanwhile make the mash. First, peel and cook the potatoes.

7 Strain the potatoes and squeeze the roasted garlic into the potatoes.

8 Mash the potatoes, mixing in the rice milk until the mash is creamy.

9 Place the veggies in a casserole dish and top with the mash.

10 Smooth with a fork and bake under the grill for a few minutes until golden brown.

WHAT YOU NEED

— 3 carrots
— 1 large onion
— 1 large leek
— 2 stalks celery
— 2–3 large floury potatoes
— 4 cloves garlic
— ½ tsp oregano
— ¾ tbsp vegetable bouillon powder
— 750 ml water
— 1 tbsp gram flour
— 2 tbsp rice milk

This dish smells sooooo good, I am certain there will be room for more!

ONE-POT STEW

HEALTH ENHANCER

Who doesn't like a tasty stew on a cold winter's evening? This one-pot wonder is chock-full of fresh veggies. It's full of flavour, functional and, believe it or not, can be made with just veggies. What more could you want? Even the meat-and-potatoes type will gobble up this scrumptious dish. Try gram flour to thicken the sauce; it's made from ground chickpeas and is available in supermarkets and health food stores – much better than bleached flour. This hearty stew is destined to become a firm family favourite.

WHAT YOU NEED

— 2 onions
— 6–8 button mushrooms
— 1 leek
— 1 small cauliflower
— 3 carrots
— 2 tbsp vegetable bouillon powder
— 750 ml water
— 10 small potatoes
— 1 tbsp gram flour

I love the wonderful aroma of this delicious stew while it's cooking, it gives me a nostalgic whiff of my mother's kitchen.

WHAT YOU DO

1 Peel and chop the vegetables into bite-size pieces.

2 Cook the onions in a pot in a small amount of water for about two minutes. Stir constantly to prevent sticking.

3 Make a stock by blending the vegetable bouillon powder with the water, and then add it to the onions.

4 Throw the veggies, potatoes, stock and herbs into the cooked onions. Bring to the boil and then reduce the heat, allowing the stew to simmer for an hour.

5 Blend the gram flour with a small amount of hot water, and then add to the stew to thicken the gravy.

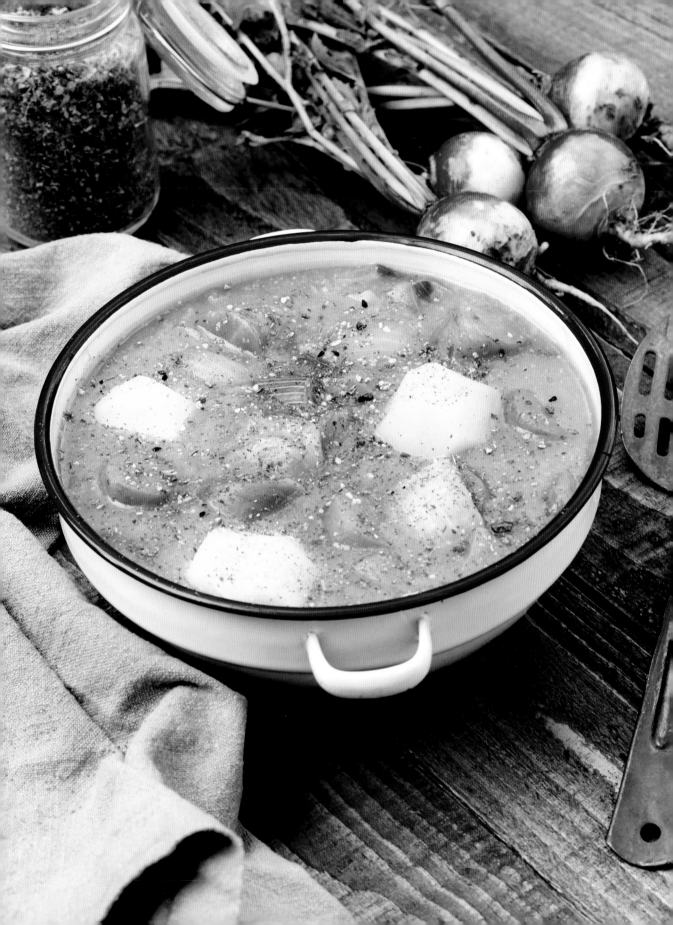

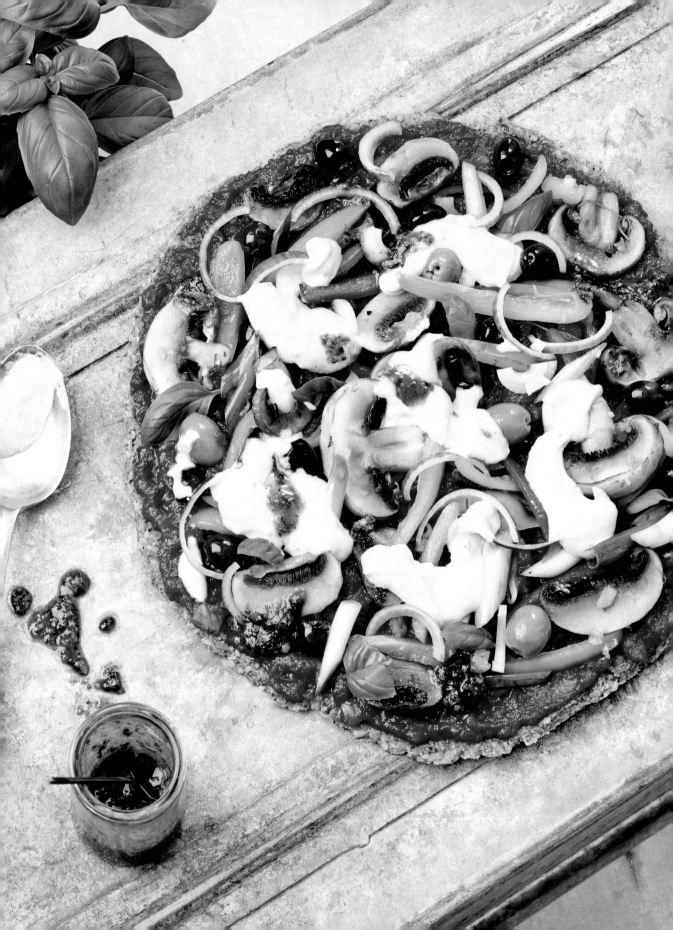

PIZZA TIME

IMMUNE BOOSTER

You may be shocked to find out that this pizza is raw. It certainly is a better option than the standard pizza that is loaded with calories and sugar. There are many ways to mimic pizza, spaghetti or lasagne. The beauty is that you can enjoy a large slice and know you are nourishing your body. Make a few crusts to save time; they will keep for two to three weeks.

The walnuts and seeds need to be soaked overnight, so you can do some of the prep the night before.

WHAT YOU DO

1 Process ingredients through a masticating juicer using the blank attachment, or alternatively process in food processor.
2 Alternate nuts, seeds and herbs to combine thoroughly.
3 Place between two sheets of parchment paper and roll out thinly.
4 Remove top sheet and place in dehydrator for 3 hours. Then turn over the crusts.
5 Continue dehydrating for 3 more hours till dry.

FAVOURITE TOPPINGS

1 Chop some of these veggies, throw them in a bowl and marinate them in garlic and olive oil for extra taste. You can choose your favourites: black olives, mushrooms, red or yellow peppers or red onion. Add fresh herbs or pesto.
2 Top the pizza bases with Sweet Pepper Sauce, page 94, your favourite toppings and No-cheese Parmigiano, page 91.
3 *Mangiate bene*, it's pizza time!

WHAT YOU NEED FOR CRUST

— *100 g walnuts, soaked overnight*
— *140 g sunflower seeds, soaked overnight*
— *180 g flax seeds, ground coarsely*
— *1 tsp Italian seasoning*
— *½ tsp dried basil*
— *½ tsp dried oregano*

When healthy food looks and tastes this good, why not eat RAW?

HOT & SPICY CURRY

IMMUNE BOOSTER

I created this curry recipe for my book *Eat Yourself Well*, and it has turned out to be one of the most popular dishes according to feedback from my readers.

To get that authentic curry flavour, this one involved many trials tweaking the amounts of spices and tons of patience. Most of the spices in this curry you will have in your spice rack. Don't forget the turmeric; besides giving food a pronounced yellow colour, it is a valued condiment that has many therapeutic benefits.

WHAT YOU NEED

— 1 onion
— 1 butternut squash
— 1 small cauliflower
— 500 ml vegetable stock
— 400 ml tin coconut milk
— 200 g yellow lentils, sprouted for two days
— 1 red chilli
— ½ tsp ginger
— 1 tsp cumin
— Pinch turmeric
— 1 tsp curry powder
— 1 tbsp gram flour

WHAT YOU DO

1 Put the onion, squash, cauliflower, chilli, ginger, cumin, turmeric and curry powder in a large pot with the vegetable stock and coconut milk.

2 Cook gently for 30 minutes, until the vegetables are soft.

3 Blend the gram flour with a small amount of hot water to thicken the sauce, and add to the pot.

4 Stir in the sprouted lentils just before serving the curry.

Keep sprouted lentils to hand to add to soups, salads and cooked meals; they are great for adding extra nutrients and vitamins to the foods you eat.

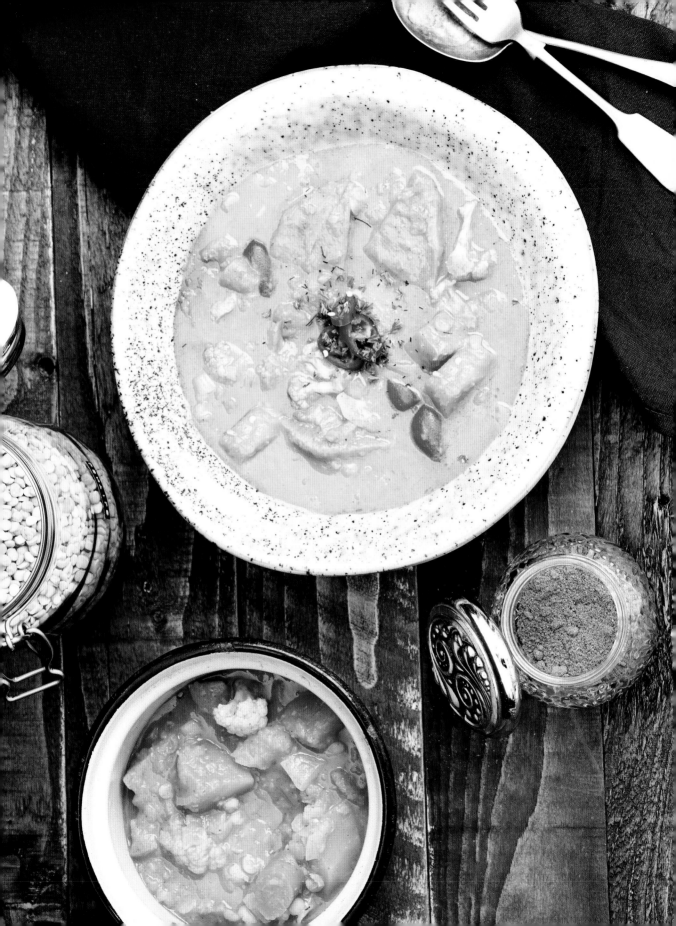

PASTA ALLA CARBONARA

IMMUNE BOOSTER

My own raw version of the Italian classic carbonara is a grain-free alternative to store-bought pasta. The best thing about this gluten-free raw pasta is that it has no empty calories, unlike the traditional stodgy pasta made from grains. Dried pasta became very popular because of its shelf life, but it's heavy and full of carbs. Courgettes are full of vitamin A, vitamin C, antioxidants, folates and potassium, and contain no saturated fats or cholesterol, unlike egg pasta.

Soak the nuts for 15 minutes beforehand to soften; this will ensure that they are nice and creamy in the sauce. Any leftovers can be served cold the next day.

WHAT YOU NEED

— *2 courgettes*
— *140 g peas*
— *½ red onion*

WHAT YOU NEED FOR SAUCE

— *30 ml lemon juice*
— *1 garlic clove*
— *70 g pine nuts*
— *140 g macadamia nuts*
— *½ tbsp pizza seasoning*
— *½ tbsp vegetable bouillon powder*

WHAT YOU DO

1 Spin the courgettes into noodles using a turning slicer and add the finely chopped red onion and peas.

2 Squash the garlic with the blade of a knife and throw all the sauce ingredients into a blender.

3 Blend till creamy and coat the veggies in the sauce. Put in a dehydrator for 10 minutes to warm slightly.

4 Top with No-cheese Parmigiano, page 91. *Buon appetito!*

If the dish gets a little dry before serving, add a few drops of olive oil and the glossy texture will be revived.

WHY &
HOW TO
SPROUT

Sprouts are by far the most nutritious whole foods on earth. I began sprouting when I was in my thirties, and I have to admit the instructions in the books I read made it seem complicated. Try as I might, I never quite managed to get it right, but even that far back in my life, I must have realised there were many benefits to be gained from this wonderful source of food that nature has provided for us. Now I teach my students how to cut through all the complicated jargon and keep the process simple and user-friendly.

Sprouts are baby plants. Let me be specific – just in case you think I am talking about Brussels sprouts – I am referring to sprouting the seeds of plants, such as alfalfa, cress, broccoli, etc. The little seedlings have a greater concentration of nutrients when the plant is starting to grow. At the two-leaf stage of growth the incredible little plants contain the most concentrated natural source of enzymes, vitamins, minerals and amino acids, which are vital for health. They have amazing healing powers and anti-cancer properties, and they cost a pittance to grow. When you sprout seeds you are basically growing your own organic foods that are free of chemicals, pesticides, herbicides and fungicides.

Start out with mung beans, lentils, alfalfa, cress or fenugreek. These are so easy to grow and will get you into the swing of sprouting. I always soak beans, lentils, nuts and seeds overnight, as it makes preparing meals the next day so fast. The only exception to this is pine nuts or macadamia nuts for quick recipes as they are softer nuts. Soaking the other seeds, beans and nuts overnight makes them more digestible and you will soon get into the habit.

Check out my favourite set of jars for sprouting (www.changesimply.com) – they have a special rack that allows the sprouts to drain completely at a 45-degree angle. This is important, as if water sits in the lid of the jar it will rot your sprouts. Remember, children grow alfalfa in eggcups in junior school, so if they can do it, so can you. It's child's play, and it takes about 5 minutes a day to produce a constant supply of these amazing, nutritious, living foods.

All you need is a set of jars, a rack, beans, seeds or nuts, and water.

WHAT TO DO FOR BEANS

1 Scoop 100 g of mung beans into a jar and cover with the lid.

2 Fill the jar with water, place the wire mesh lid on the jar and soak overnight.

3 Drain the water and rinse under a tap. Place the jar upside down on a rack at a 45-degree angle to allow the water to drain completely.

4 Rinse once a day for 2 or 3 days. In warmer climates, rinsing twice a day works best.

5 When the roots begin to emerge from the beans they are ready to eat. Store in the refrigerator to extend the shelf life of your sprouts to 5 or 6 days.

WHAT TO DO FOR SEEDS

1 Basically, it's exactly the same procedure, except you need a smaller quantity of seeds – about 25 g per jar should do it.

WHAT TO DO FOR NUTS

1 Nuts don't really sprout, but they should be soaked and rinsed to make them more digestible.

2 Put the desired amount of nuts into a jar and cover with the lid. Fill the jar with water and soak overnight. Drain the water and rinse under a tap.

3 Place the jar upside down on the rack at a 45-degree angle to allow the water to drain completely.

4 The nuts are then ready for use.

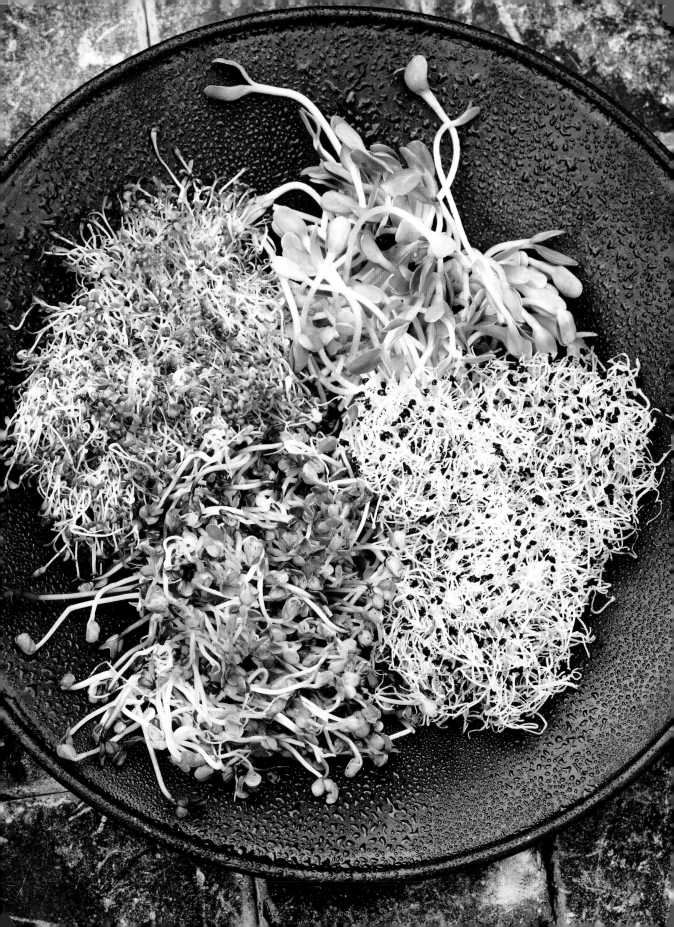

'Never eat more than you can lift.'
MISS PIGGY

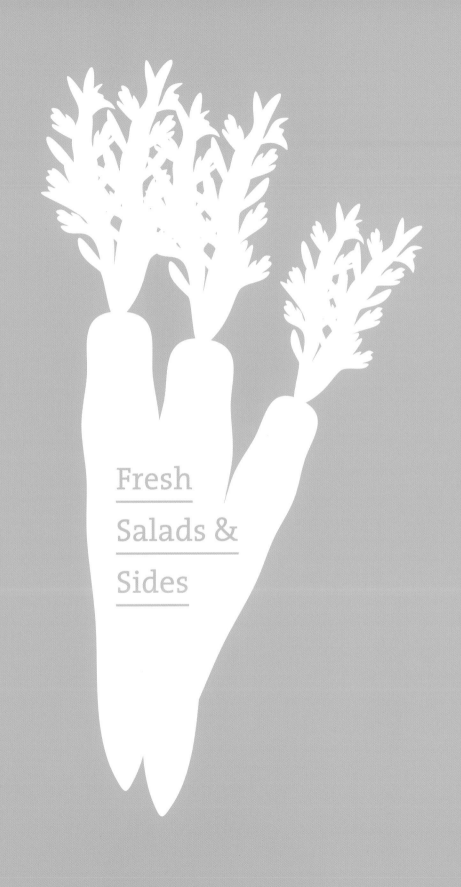

Fresh
Salads &
Sides

When you are preparing food, why not make something that will actually nourish your body? You don't have to be deprived to eat healthily. You might think you will be missing out when eating raw foods, or that it's some extreme and boring way of eating, but it's not. This is real food that nourishes your body, not the fake stuff that damages it. What you will miss out on are the fried, calorie-loaded, factory-created processed foods that are full of chemical preservatives. In my opinion, that is an absolute advantage of a raw diet, not a drawback.

If others scoff at or dismiss your choice of opting for the raw food lifestyle, think of the athletes and celebrities who focus big-time on their physical appearance, and have attributed their slim figures and glowing looks to eating raw foods. Nowadays, there is huge media attention paid to the dietary habits of celebrities, and those who have embraced the raw food lifestyle in some form include Pierce Brosnan, Demi Moore, Cher, Susan Sarandon, Daryl Hannah, Scarlett Johansson, Rosanna Davison and pro Ironman triathlete Brendan Brazier, to name a few.

I hope the array of delicious choices that are now as close as the turn of a page away will convince you that you can relish a meal and satisfy your palate with raw, nutritious foods. You can trade in the greasy take-away for a yummy 'stir-raw' with low-carb rice, or pair Carb-free Spaghetti with a Sweet Pepper Pasta Sauce and crumble a nice raw cheese on top. Trust me, you won't miss the junk. It will soon become a walk in the park and you will be whipping up raw meals in a flash.

Remember it's not all or nothing – just do your best. To make the transition smooth, have a juice for breakfast and a scrumptious, inviting salad for lunch or dinner. Spruce up a salad by using different food preparation techniques to add interesting textures. A vegetable spiraliser comes in handy for making raw spaghetti, vegetable noodles, chips or fine shoestring garnishes.

Avocados can give soups, smoothies, dressings, dips and desserts a fabulous creamy texture. They are rich in omega-3 fatty acids and vitamin E, which is great for your skin and hair.

Mushrooms are also a great addition to vegetarian or vegan dishes as they give a chewy texture, which is very satisfying. Some mushrooms are also a rich source of vitamin D, which is necessary for absorbing calcium. Flavouring is very important for any food, whether cooked or raw, so add fresh herbs, spices and seasonings to your raw food meals. These recipes will help you embrace eating nourishing food even within a busy schedule.

CUCUMBER, AVOCADO & RAW MAYO

IMMUNE BOOSTER

Full of healthful compounds, this refreshing salad is bursting with flavour, and it's so easy to prepare. The mayo blends beautifully with the creamy texture of the avocados. Cucumbers contain a host of vitamins: vitamin B1, vitamin B2, vitamin B3, vitamin B5, vitamin B6, folic acid, vitamin C, calcium, iron, magnesium, phosphorus, potassium and zinc. Cucumbers contain enough sugar and electrolytes to replenish essential nutrients and keep you hydrated.

WHAT YOU NEED

— 1 cucumber, very thinly sliced
— ½ small red onion, thinly sliced
— 2 ripe avocados, peeled, destoned and diced

WHAT YOU NEED FOR RAW MAYO

— 125 ml water
— 60 ml olive oil
— 140 g organic raw pine nuts, soaked for 15 minutes
— 50 g raw cauliflower
— 2 tbsp lemon juice
— 1 tsp yellow mustard
— Handful chopped mint

WHAT YOU DO

1 Slice the cucumber and red onion thinly, and then dice the avocado.
2 Whisk together the mayo ingredients to a creamy consistency. Adjust to taste.
3 Add the cucumber and onion, and coat the vegetables with the mayo mixture.
4 Add the avocado last, and stir to coat.
5 Garnish with some chopped mint.

This mayo makes a fantastic dressing for coleslaw or a sandwich spread.

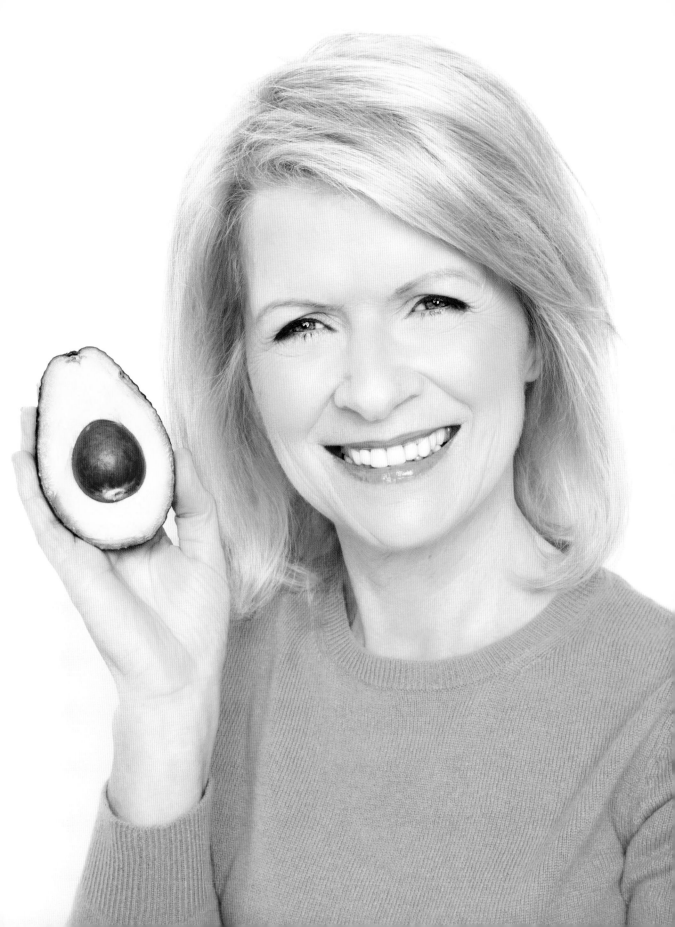

FEEL-GREAT SPROUTED SALAD

IMMUNE BOOSTER

Sprouted seeds are packed with nutrition and are very much part of my daily diet. They are extremely cheap to produce and are great value for money, particularly when you consider their many benefits. They improve the immune system, help the body to flush out waste, and they also protect us against disease. Simply throw some lemon juice, garlic, fresh herbs and freshly grated ginger together for an explosion of crunchy, fragrant nourishment.

WHAT YOU NEED

— *2 handfuls sprouted seeds (alfalfa, onion, sunflower or broccoli)*
— *Handful basil*
— *1 red onion*
— *1 red pepper*
— *1 carrot, grated*
— *35 g pine nuts*

WHAT YOU DO

1 Slice the onion and red pepper, and grate the carrot.

2 Toss your chosen sprouts into the mix and add the pine nuts.

3 Drizzle with your favourite dressing. How simple is that?

Not only are sprouts super-foods, their visual appeal is a wonderful boost to any salad or sandwich.

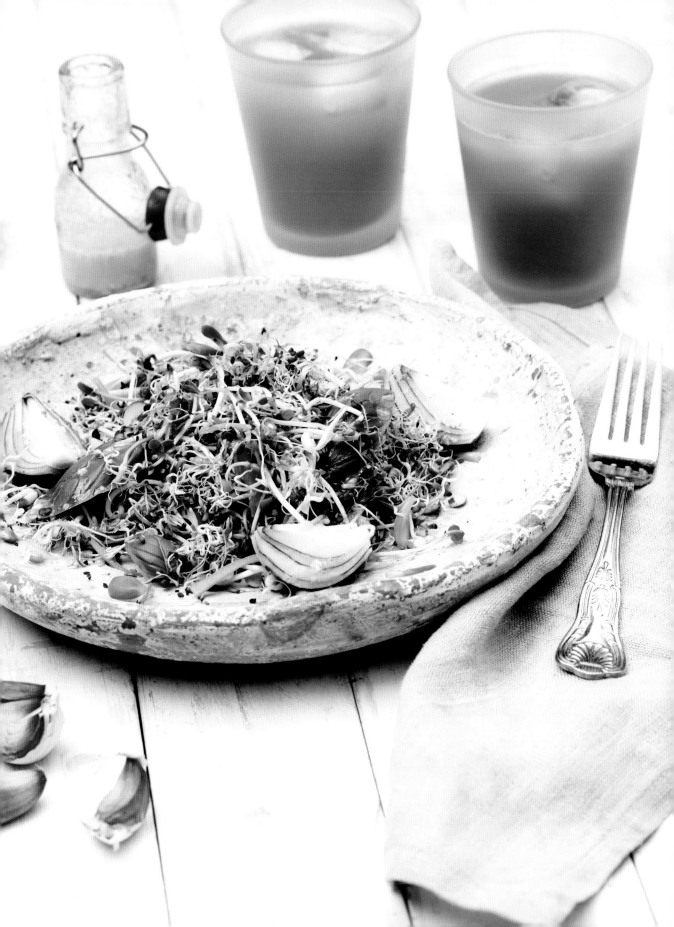

ZESTY SPROUTED SALAD

IMMUNE BOOSTER

Sprouting beans is the best way to eat legumes if you want to make them more digestible. It's well worth the small amount of time and effort it takes when you consider that the proteins, vitamins and minerals in legumes quadruple when they are sprouted. Mung beans have anti-cancer properties, and are said to stop premature ageing. I find it hard to get fresh coconut, so I use a can of coconut milk. When I open it, I scoop off the thick coconut from the top, pat it dry with kitchen paper and chop into little pieces. Keep the remaining coconut water for smoothies.

WHAT YOU NEED

— *2 handfuls sprouted mung beans*
— *½ cucumber*
— *½ red pepper*
— *2 carrots*
— *juice of 1 lime*
— *1 tbsp oil*
— *1 tbsp coconut pieces*
— *½ small red chilli pepper*
— *celery salt to taste*

This unassuming salad is chock-full of zest, and is quick, mega nutritious and refreshing.

WHAT YOU DO

1   Sprout and rinse the mung beans thoroughly. Pat dry before adding to the salad to remove the excess water.
2   Slice the cucumber, red pepper and carrots thinly.
3   Scoop off the thick coconut from the top of the tin of coconut milk, pat it dry with kitchen paper and chop into little pieces. Finely dice the chilli.
4   Add the mung beans to the salad and combine.
5   Blend the oil, lime, garlic and celery salt together, pour over the salad and season.
6   Top with the chopped coconut and serve.

ANTI-INFLAMMATORY SALAD

IMMUNE BOOSTER

Traditionally, beetroot was eaten for its anti-inflammatory properties. It is a strong antioxidant that is high in fibre and iron. Beetroot is also rich in silica, which is good for our skin, connective tissues and bone health. It is much more beneficial to eat raw beetroot as the oxalic acid becomes harmful when cooked. I never juice beets as they are loaded with sugars, but the green leaves can be juiced.

WHAT YOU DO

1 Juice the lemon.
2 Peel the ginger and throw all the ingredients into a blender.
3 Serve as a side with a fresh green salad.

WHAT YOU NEED

— *1 beetroot*
— *¼-inch piece ginger*
— *Juice of 1 lemon*

This salad will tickle your taste buds. The alkalizing lemon is perfect with the beetroot and ginger; they make a lovely healthy combo.

CAESAR SALAD WITH CREAMY DRESSING

IMMUNE BOOSTER

A classic Caesar salad is usually made with anchovies, which, I admit, make me squeamish. To replace the fishy flavour, I have used hijiki seaweed, a wild seaweed that grows on rocky coastlines around Japan. You can buy it in supermarkets and health stores. If you don't have hijiki seaweed, you can sprinkle the salad with dulse flakes.

WHAT YOU NEED FOR SALAD

— *1 head iceberg lettuce*
— *20 g hijiki seaweed*
— *1 small red onion*

WHAT YOU NEED FOR DRESSING

— *100 g pine nuts*
— *5 basil leaves*
— *1 tbsp nutritional yeast*
— *1 clove garlic*
— *pinch celery salt*
— *60 ml olive oil*
— *Juice of 4 limes*

WHAT YOU DO

1 Soak the seaweed in water for 30 minutes while you make the dressing and prepare the salad.
2 Drain the seaweed and pat it with a paper towel.
3 Blend the ingredients for the dressing.
4 Shave the onion thinly and toss the lettuce, seaweed and dressing together.

Crisp iceberg lettuce with shaved red onion in a scrumptious dressing, topped with No-cheese Parmigiano (p. 91).

DILL-ICIOUSLY STUFFED PEPPERS

IMMUNE BOOSTER

Dill and lemon mingle well in this *dill-icious* dish; the sharpness of the lemon balances beautifully with the fresh herb. If you are not eating as many veggies as you would like to, try this and get all the benefits of the nutritious ingredients. Bragg Liquid Aminos is excellent for quick marinades – you simply add it to some oil. These stuffed peppers are a satisfying filler for hungry tummies; you will be stuffed too.

WHAT YOU DO

1 Wash and cut the peppers in half and discard the seeds.
2 Marinate in liquid aminos and oil for 20 minutes, turning occasionally.

WHAT YOU DO FOR STUFFING

1 Process in a blender the nuts, lemon, avocado, sweetcorn, bouillon, onion and dill, adding the oil last. Process to a chunky consistency.
2 Stuff each pepper evenly with the mixture.
3 Place in dehydrator for 1 hour 30 minutes.

WHAT YOU NEED

— *1 red pepper*
— *1 yellow pepper*
— *60 ml Bragg Liquid Aminos*
— *60 ml olive oil*

WHAT YOU NEED FOR STUFFING

— *50 g walnuts*
— *1 avocado*
— *90 g sweetcorn*
— *1 small onion*
— *½ tsp vegetable bouillon*
— *1 tbsp olive oil*
— *Few sprigs fresh dill*
— *Juice of ½ lemon*

OMEGA-RICH WRAPS

IMMUNE BOOSTER

This is the ultimate quick-fix lunch. It can be pulled together in minutes for those moments when you are ready to eat the leg off of the table. Avocados are full of monounsaturated fats that help increase good cholesterol (HDL) and reduce the bad stuff (LDL). They are also loaded with vitamin C, vitamin K, B6, folate and are high in fibre. A lot of sambos these days are full of processed junk and they also contain lashings of salt.

These wraps are super quick, tasty and mega healthy.

WHAT YOU NEED

— 4 lettuce leaves
— 2 avocados
— 1 carrot
— ½ red pepper
— ½ cucumber
— 1 small red onion
— Handful alfalfa sprouts
— 2 tsp garlic oil
— 1 tsp lemon juice
— Pinch cayenne pepper

WHAT YOU DO

1 Chop cucumber, red pepper and carrot into matchsticks. Dice the red onion.
2 Mash the avocados with lemon juice, garlic oil, cayenne pepper and add the diced red onion.
3 Fill each lettuce leaf with the sprouts and match-stick veggies.
4 Add ¼ of the avocado mix to each leaf and wrap the leaves together.

The healthy fats in avocados help to sustain you throughout the day so you can avoid the dreaded afternoon slump.

QUICK PARSNIP RICE

IMMUNE BOOSTER

Preparing proper, homemade dinners can be a challenge, especially if you are zapped after a long day. No matter how hectic your lifestyle, you have to eat food to fuel your body. This simple, time-saving dish can be served with a nice green salad or a 'stir-raw'. There is great joy in exploring new tastes and taking the boredom out of preparing food. Pine nuts are quite oily and give the dish a fried rice effect when dehydrated. Rice has very little taste of its own; it's the sauce you add or the food you serve with it that adds flavour. Unlike ordinary rice, you won't have to watch the pot.

WHAT YOU DO

1 Peel the parsnips and place, with the nuts and oil, in a processor and chop finely.
2 Place on parchment paper in a dehydrator until warm (approximately 2 to 10 minutes) and serve.

WHAT YOU NEED

— *2 parsnips*
— *70 g pine nuts, soaked*
— *2 tsp olive oil*

I was never a lover of parsnips, but I find they work well in this dish. You can also use cauliflower if you prefer.

GARLIC SWEET POTATO MASH

IMMUNE BOOSTER

If you are looking for culinary inspiration, why not reawaken your taste buds with some different flavours and tastes? I know only too well that there is no joy in spending hours in your kitchen, preparing food that finicky eaters turn their noses up at. When you are trying to get the family on board, you need to make food tasty and interesting. I promise this sweet, tasty mash will get the thumbs up.

WHAT YOU NEED

— *3 sweet potatoes, peeled and cubed*
— *1 tbsp garlic oil*
— *Pinch cayenne pepper*
— *Few sprigs parsley (optional)*
— *Pinch celery salt*

My Julie is obsessed with this – she is always licking the spoon and coming back for more.

WHAT YOU DO

1 Boil the sweet potatoes in water until tender and drain.

2 Add the garlic oil and mash until smooth and creamy.

3 Add celery salt and a pinch of cayenne pepper to taste.

4 Garnish with parsley, if you are a fan of it.

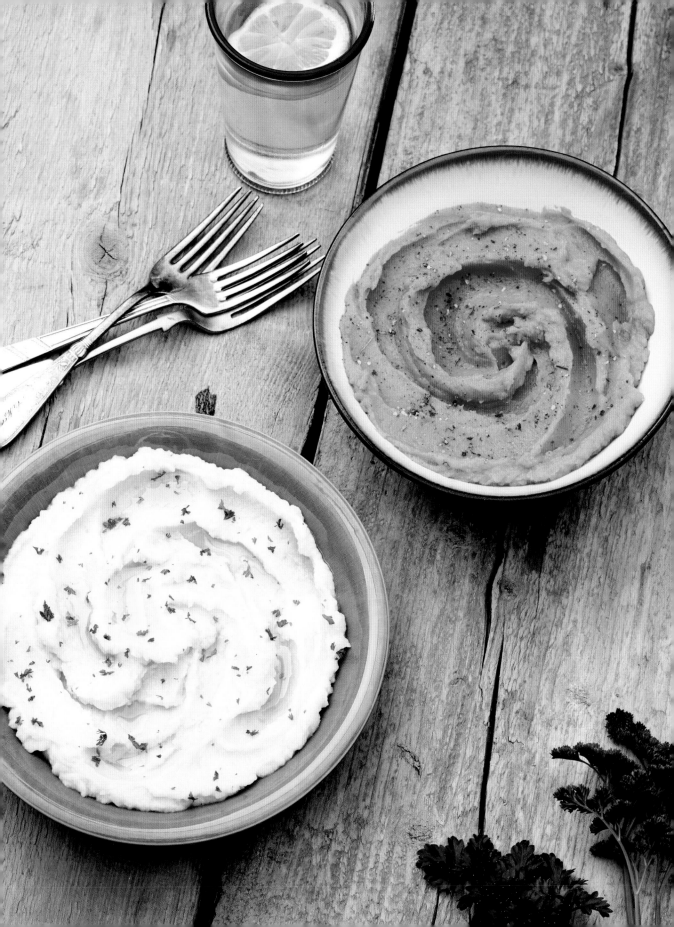

LOW-CARB GARLIC MASH

IMMUNE BOOSTER

This is a great addition to any meal – you can serve it with salads or roast vegetables. It's a good low-carb alternative to plain old potatoes, which as I already mentioned can be a problem for those with joint pains. Potatoes are nightshades, and include a substance called alkaloids, which can have a negative impact on joints and nerve and muscle function. So, if you have arthritic problems, they may not be the best food for you. I like to use garlic-infused olive oil to make a nice creamy mash. You can make your own garlic oil, but most stores also stock it. A delicious mash that contains no heart-clogging butter.

WHAT YOU NEED

— 1 large cauliflower
— 2 tsp garlic olive oil
— 2 spring onions
— Pinch cayenne pepper
— Pinch celery salt

This mash has been a big hit with my friends and students not only for its taste, but because it is so easy to prepare.

WHAT YOU DO

1 Wash the cauliflower and chop the spring onions.
2 Steam the cauliflower till tender. Then place the steamed cauliflower in a processor and drizzle with oil.
3 Blend till thick and creamy. Add the chopped spring onions, cayenne pepper and celery salt to taste, and serve immediately.

IMMUNE-BOOSTING SPINACH

IMMUNE BOOSTER

Spinach is a great immune-booster that provides important nutrients for the eyes and skin. I love baby spinach as it's so versatile; you can throw it into juices, smoothies, salads and it is ideal for this delicious creamed spinach. It's important to buy organic spinach because the leaf tends to be heavily sprayed with pesticides that you can't wash off.

I sometimes use up the pulp that is left over from nut milk to thicken this dish. I dehydrate the pulp till dry, and place it in a jar until I am ready to use it. If you don't have almond pulp, top with No-cheese Parmigiano, page 91.

WHAT YOU DO

1 Combine all the ingredients apart from the spinach in the blender.
2 Add the spinach to mixture and blend till combined.
3 Top with No-cheese Parmigiano, page 91 (optional).

WHAT YOU NEED

— 450 g baby spinach
— 200 g pine nuts
— Juice of 1 lemon
— 1 tsp nutritional yeast
— ½ tsp onion powder
— 1 garlic clove
— 190 ml coconut milk
— Celery salt to taste

Using coconut milk instead of dairy adds an exotic appeal to this luscious, creamy dish.

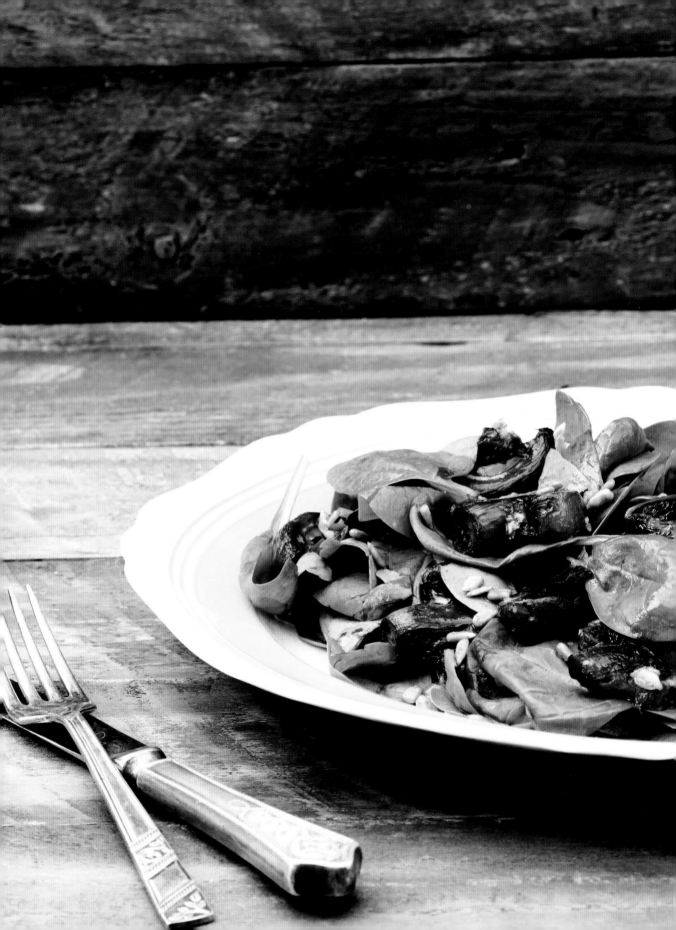

SPINACH SALAD WITH GARLIC MUSHROOMS

IMMUNE BOOSTER

Mushrooms are loaded with B vitamins and add a chewy texture to dishes. What a great, simple salad. You dehydrate the mushrooms in oil and garlic and, *voilà*, you're done. They smell delicious and taste even better.

WHAT YOU DO

1. Clean and slice the mushrooms.
2. Crush the garlic cloves and mix with the oil in a bowl.
3. Add the mushrooms to the oil mix and allow them to soak it up.
4. Dehydrate for 30–40 minutes.
5. Wash the baby spinach leaves and top with mushrooms. Drizzle with your favourite dressing if desired.

WHAT YOU NEED

— *400 g mushrooms*
— *3 garlic cloves*
— *100 ml extra virgin olive oil*
— *200 g baby spinach*

Yes, I know I use a lot of spinach, but it's so good for you.

'A human being
has a natural desire to
have more of a good
thing than he needs.'
MARK TWAIN

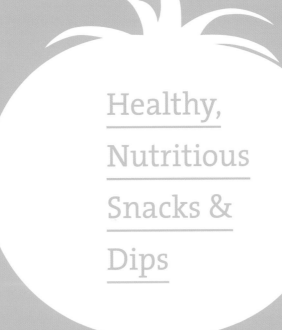

Healthy,
Nutritious
Snacks &
Dips

Producing family-friendly healthy recipes has become a passion for me. I have taught in schools to children, teens and parents about the foods best able to promote children's health. In fact, with the arrival of my first grandchild, Ella, who has changed the course of my life in many wonderful ways, and the numerous mums who have sent so many photos of their kids drinking green juice, munching sprouts and even drinking wheat grass, it has fuelled my passion all the more. I feel blessed to be able to help these mums build strong healthy bodies and improve the foods their children eat in the home and at school.

Despite the fact that it is vitally important to sustain our children's health and well-being, it can be difficult, especially if you are battling between the stove and Lego. That's family life nowadays; we are always on the run, but if we want to reverse the epidemic of childhood obesity, early-onset diabetes and ADHD in our children and teens, we need to encourage healthy eating habits from the beginning. If your cupboards are full of junk food that they can snack on, then that is exactly what will happen. A fussy toddler sometimes needs to be hungry in order to eat proper meals.

It's easy to get children to eat healthily if you know how, and what better way to do this than making your own delicious, nutritious snacks. I became quite sneaky with my teenagers and managed to sneak quite a lot of healthy stuff into meals in not-too-obvious ways, which was a necessary strategy that helped them to adjust. I used this tactic with my teenagers rather than doing battle every night of the week, and it worked. I added essential fats to smoothies and mashed potatoes, spinach and probiotics into smoothies and all kinds of veggies to juices without complaint. This simple tactic changed the way they ate. Needs must!

Ideally, it's better to set a good example, as parents are their child's greatest role models and they depend on you to provide a healthy attitude towards food. I am a massive believer that the essential ingredient for good health is education. It helps you make informed decisions, but this does not always work with a fussy toddler or grumpy teenager. Your efforts to improve their health may cause conflict at meal times.

My greatest joy was with our then five-year-old daughter Julie, who was still at an age where it was easy to influence her eating habits. Her enthusiasm was infectious, and I encouraged her all the way. I taught her which foods helped the different parts of her body, as she whisked a sauce or stirred a pot. We found lots of products that were good alternatives: for example, for cow's milk, we substituted rice or almond milk. Sugar we substituted with stevia, and dairy butter with almond or hazelnut butter. Julie is now 20 years old; thankfully, she has never

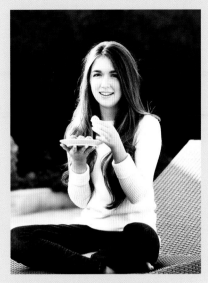

had an antibiotic in her life. Her slim figure, long shiny hair and glowing skin say it all. Her health on the inside shines on the outside.

Remember, if I can do it, so can you. Try making your own crisps, they really are delicious. If this sounds difficult or time-consuming, well, believe me, you don't need to be a master chef by any stretch. They are packed with flavour and will be enjoyed by all. You will need to invest in a small dehydrator, which is an inexpensive food-drying machine (see page 15 for more details). I promise it's worth the investment for the crisps alone. It's so economical to make your own nutritious snacks, and there are no added preservatives or harmful oils used in the process. You can also make biscuits, crackers and main meals that will produce satisfying, tasty and enzyme-rich foods for yourself and your family.

Put the crisps in a bowl in an accessible spot, and you will find sneaky hands soon gobble them up. I usually make a few trays of kale crisps over the weekend hoping they will last the week, but my gang soon demolish the lot.

Best of luck!

CRACKERS ABOUT CRACKERS

IMMUNE BOOSTER

Onions are wonderful for the prevention and treatment of many common diseases such as cancer, coronary heart disease and diabetes. They are amazingly rich in sulforaphanes, a group of phytochemicals, which are disease-fighting compounds found in plant-based foods.

Most store-bought crackers contain hidden sugars and hydrogenated fats. When you make your own, you know exactly what you're eating. Flax seeds are a good source of omega-3 fatty acids; they are also rich in fibre and proteins.

WHAT YOU NEED

— 2 stalks celery
— 1 white onion
— 1 clove garlic
— 180 g flax seeds
— 140 g sunflower seeds
— 60 ml Bragg Liquid Aminos
— 60 ml olive oil
— ½ red chilli, finely chopped
— ½ tsp celery salt
— 500 ml water

You cannot compare the delicious taste of home-made crackers with the store-bought varieties.

WHAT YOU DO

1   Soak the sunflower and flax seeds (separately) in a cup of water overnight.
2   Rinse off the sunflower seeds, but use all of the gelatinous flax seed mix.
3   Peel the onions and wash the celery, and chop them finely in a processor.
4   Mix with the remaining ingredients until completely combined.
5   Spread the mixture thinly over two sheets of parchment. Sprinkle with celery salt.
6   Score into the mixture with a pizza cutter to make square or rectangular shapes.
7   Dehydrate overnight. If the crackers are not fully dry, return them to the dehydrator until drying is complete.

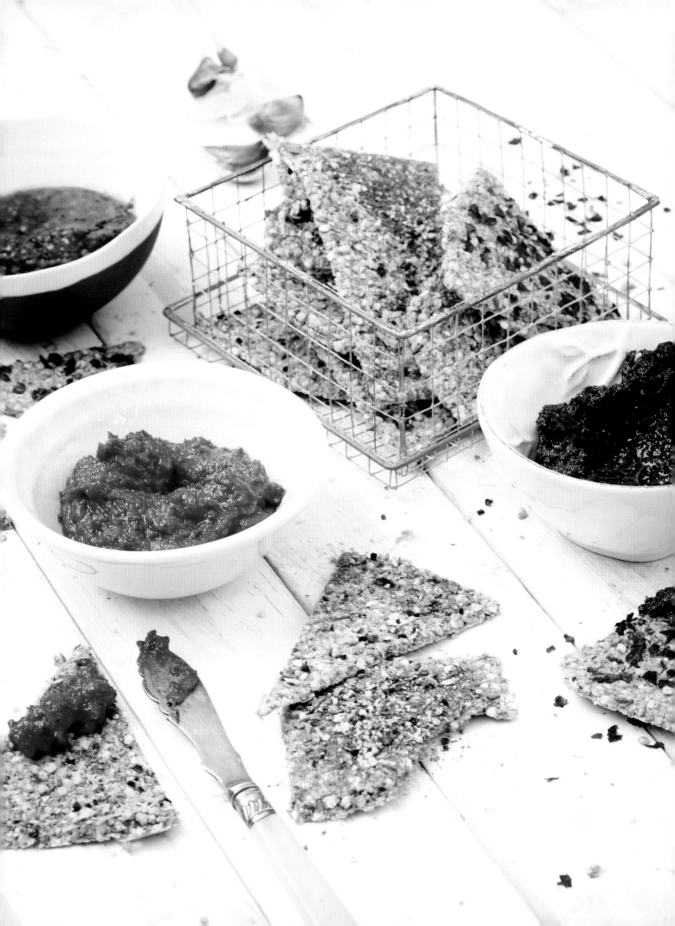

HEART-FRIENDLY PESTO

IMMUNE BOOSTER

Pesto makes a nice change to stir into pasta than the typical tomato-based sauces. I love it drizzled over salads or on crackers. Pine nuts are rich in vitamin C and heart-friendly monounsaturated fats – plus, here I have added some extra good fats with the Udo's oil to up your intake of good fats. The nutritional yeast in this recipe gives the pesto that cheesy taste.

WHAT YOU NEED

— *1 bunch fresh basil*
— *140 g pine nuts*
— *1 clove garlic*
— *1–2 tbsp Udo's oil*
— *Juice of ½ a lemon*
— *1 tsp nutritional yeast*

WHAT YOU DO

1 Process all the ingredients except the Udo's oil.
2 Gradually drizzle in the oil until the pesto turns to a rough paste.

Homemade pesto tastes nothing like the ready-made stuff you buy in a jar. Go on, give it a go.

LOVELY TAPENADE

IMMUNE BOOSTER

I am in love with the simplicity of this tapenade. You don't know how hard it is for me not to scoff all of it when I make a bowl; but then, I am a lover of olives and basil.

It's quite salty as olives are high in sodium; however, they are also a good source of healthy fats. This pungent mush is great for nibbles, tapas or hors d'œuvres at a party. Pitted olives are more convenient and save time if you are looking for something quick.

WHAT YOU DO

1 Process all ingredients into a rough paste before gradually adding the olive oil. Yum, yum!

WHAT YOU NEED

— *140 g black olives*
— *1 clove garlic*
— *2 tbsp olive oil*
— *¼ tsp Dijon mustard*

Tapenade is traditionally made in a pestle and mortar, but nowadays you can whizz it up in a blender.

RED PEPPER SALSA

IMMUNE BOOSTER

This salsa is incredibly easy and certainly packs a punch. If you like spicy salsa, add the full red chilli. It will keep for a week in the fridge without growing hairy stuff. Although after a week it may still look okay to eat, nutritionally it will not be so good as the enzymes will have been lost.

I like it really fresh and juicy when the peppers are straight from the farmer's market.

WHAT YOU NEED

— 1 red pepper
— 1 small red onion
— Juice of ½ a lemon
— ½ tsp celery salt
— ½ red chilli
— 1–2 tbsp olive oil
— 2 tbsp dried parsley or basil

WHAT YOU DO

1 De-seed the red pepper and chilli.
2 Chop all remaining ingredients coarsely in a blender.

Serve it with crackers and parsnip crisps.

SMOKED CHIPOTLE HUMMUS

IMMUNE BOOSTER

I've eaten my fair share of this popular Middle Eastern dip, and I always have a good supply in the fridge. Hummus is a great standby to have on hand. I like to sprinkle some smoked chipotle chilli powder to give this hummus a kick, but if you don't like spicy food you can omit the dried chilli powder. I have used tinned chickpeas in this recipe, but you can use dried chickpeas to make a raw hummus with sprouted chickpeas if you want to stay raw.

Be warned, dust gently with the chipotle powder – you don't want to burn your mouth. If you overdo it and add too much, don't panic, you can always scoop it off.

WHAT YOU DO

1   Place all the ingredients in a food processor, except the chipotle powder.
2   Blend into a smooth mix.
3   Swirl on a drizzle of Udo's oil before serving and dust with the smoked dried chilli powder, if desired.

WHAT YOU NEED

— *1 garlic clove, crushed*
— *240 g tinned chickpeas, drained*
— *2 tbsp tahini (sesame seed paste)*
— *Juice of ½ a lemon*
— *2 tbsp Udo's oil*
— *Pinch smoked chipotle chilli powder (optional)*

This spicy hummus keeps for three days in the fridge.

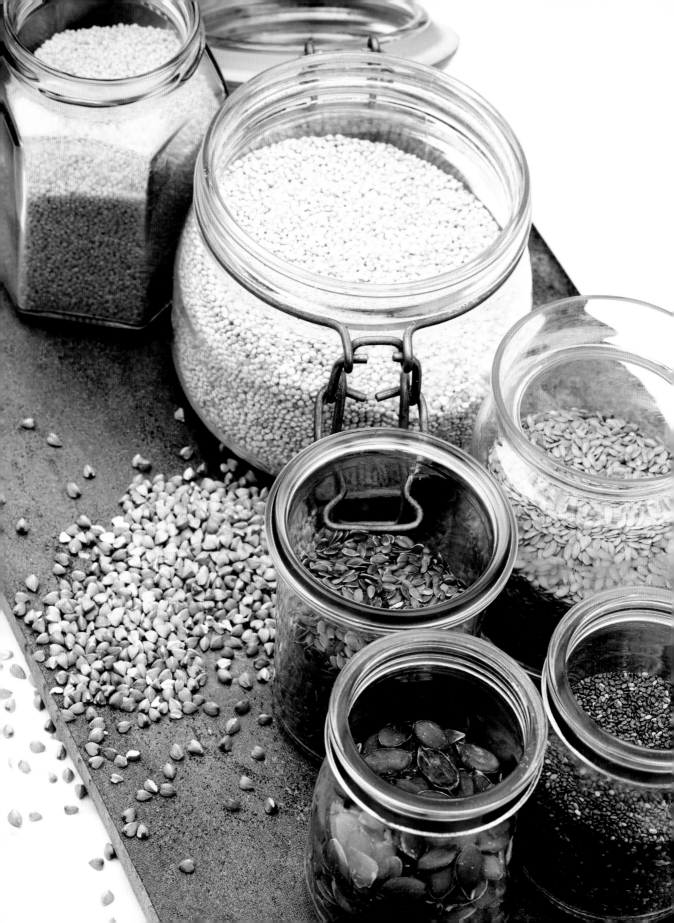

GOOD & CRUNCHY SEED SNACKS

Sprouted seeds are so full of goodness that they are a must in your diet. Sprout sunflower seeds, pumpkin seeds or sesame seeds for rich sources of proteins, antioxidants, vitamin E, calcium, fibre and essential fats. When you sprout the seeds they are more digestible, and they give you a steady flow of energy throughout the day. Sprout for one day, coat them in your favourite herbs and spices and dehydrate to intensify the flavour.

WHAT YOU DO

1 Sprout the seeds in water overnight and drain thoroughly.
2 Mix the seasonings in a bowl and throw in the sprouted seeds. Coat the seeds in the seasoning mix.
3 Spread seed mixture on parchment paper and dehydrate till dry. Store in a glass jar.

WHAT YOU NEED

— *2 tbsp sunflower seeds*
— *35 g sesame seeds*
— *45 g pumpkin seeds*
— *2 tsp Bragg Liquid Aminos*
— *½ tsp celery salt*
— *Pinch curry powder*
— *2 tsp olive oil*

You can create your own mix of spices, with chilli, curry, wasabi, ginger, cardamom, turmeric, cumin or cayenne pepper, and have some creative fun in the kitchen.

AMAZING CRACKERS

IMMUNE BOOSTER

The salty seaweed is a perfect match with the cheesy taste of the nutritional yeast. If you are watching your waistline, or trying to avoid the high calories found in commercial crackers, these amazing crackers are a healthy option. With a lovely crunchy texture, they work really well with hummus and dips. You can also spread them with avocado or tapenade, or simply eat them with your favourite salad.

Cumin seeds have a nutty, peppery taste and they are a key ingredient of curry powder. Cumin is rich in iron, which is a vital component of haemoglobin. It's also rich in calcium, manganese and magnesium. It slows down free-radical damage in the body, and research shows it has anti-cancer effects.

I like to add cumin to crackers; this spice gives a good kick to crackers, soups and sauces. I use the seed rather than cumin powder, as the seeds can be easily ground with a mortar and pestle, and they don't lose their flavour as quickly as the powder.

Make sure you buy nuts in smallish quantities, as they can go rancid.

WHAT YOU NEED

— 4 nori seaweed sheets
— 200 g walnuts, soaked
— 1 red pepper
— 1 stick celery
— 100 g nutritional yeast
— Pinch smoked chipotle powder
— 1 tsp smoked paprika
— 1 tsp ground cumin
— 250 ml water

WHAT YOU DO

1 Combine all the ingredients in a blender.
2 Add a little water to blend into a dough-like consistency.
3 Adjust the flavouring to suit your taste.
4 Spread onto parchment paper and score square shapes into the dough. This makes it easy to break the crackers when they are dry.
5 Dehydrate overnight until dry and crispy.

These crackers are amazing!

LIP-SMACKING ONION CRISPS

IMMUNE BOOSTER

When you need something to munch on, don't reach for crisps that are fried and heated in oils, as they have a terrible impact on our health. Heating oils at high temperatures changes their structure into twisted molecules called trans-fatty acids. Fried fats cause a hardening of the arteries and make blood platelets sticky. They increase the danger of free-radical damage, and may cause pathogenic problems.

WHAT YOU DO

1 Blend the sweetcorn and vegetable bouillon together until it forms a creamy batter.

2 Add some water to the batter if it is too thick; make it the consistency of a pancake batter.

3 Slice the onions into fairly thick rings and coat the onions rings in the batter.

4 Place the coated onions rings on a dehydrator tray and dry till crisp, turning once.

WHAT YOU NEED

— *3 white onions*
— *350 g frozen sweetcorn*
— *1 tbsp reduced-salt vegetable bouillon*
— *250 ml water*

If the idea of making your own crisps doesn't light your fire, maybe you think it's too difficult. Let me tell you, it's not! Come on, give it a try.

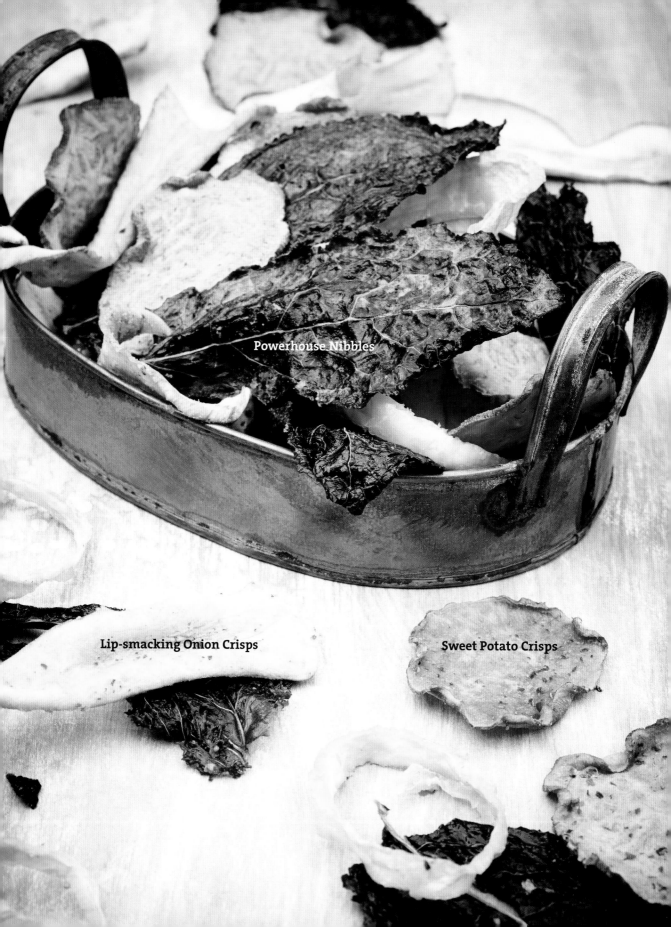

Powerhouse Nibbles

Lip-smacking Onion Crisps

Sweet Potato Crisps

POWERHOUSE NIBBLES

IMMUNE BOOSTER

This is a pretty awesome snack that will not only stave off the munchies, but is also an excellent source of nutrients, especially vitamin A, beta-carotene and calcium. Kale is high in fibre, which helps to create the bulk you need to fill you up, and is one of the most nutritious vegetables out there.

These crisps can be prepared in a flash, but take some time to dehydrate. They are packed full of flavour and nutrients. You can buy some of these crisps in speciality stores, but it is much more economical to make your own.

WHAT YOU DO

1 Remove the kale from its stalks. Don't waste these, keep them to add to a juice later.
2 Combine the oil and the veggie bouillon. Lightly coat the kale in the mixture and place on the dehydrator tray. Don't be afraid to get your hands dirty. Stir with your hands, rubbing the mix into the kale as you go.
3 Dry until crisp, turning once during the drying process.

WHAT YOU NEED

— *1 bunch kale*
— *1 tbsp vegetable bouillon*
— *125 ml olive oil*

Kale can be added to side dishes, main dishes or salads, but it's absolutely fabulous for these crisps.

SNACK ATTACK

IMMUNE BOOSTER

When you are a crisp addict, sometimes you will stop at nothing to get your fix. These crisps are great when you get a snack attack. Turmeric gives these crisps their pronounced yellow colour; it's a valued condiment that adds flavour but also has amazing healing properties. I never use the centre of the parsnip as it is too tough for crisps, but I make the no-carb rice from the leftovers. I find that the minute these crisps are prepared, they disappear quickly, especially when my son Richard is around.

WHAT YOU NEED

— 2 parsnips
— 1 tbsp vegetable bouillon
— ¼ tsp onion powder
— Pinch turmeric
— 375 ml hot water

This is a scrummy snack that you won't feel guilty about scoffing.

WHAT YOU DO

1 Mix the bouillon, onion powder and turmeric with hot water.
2 Slice the parsnips thinly and dip in seasoning mix.
3 Place on dehydrator tray.
4 Dry until crisp, turning once during the drying process.

S.O.S. CRISPS

IMMUNE BOOSTER

When you're trying to stick to your healthy lifestyle, you may be tempted by your favourite cheese and onion, salt and vinegar, spicy tortilla, prawn cocktail, barbecue or balsamic vinegar crisps – and once you start, you will not be able to stop. We eat a whopping 5 billion packets of crisps a year. It's pretty obvious that we have an unhealthy appetite for crisps of all kinds, and they're very unhealthy: fried in fat, covered in salt and heart-clogging. These S.O.S. crisps are great to have at hand for emergencies. They will come to the rescue and are the perfect healthy solution.

WHAT YOU DO

1 Blend the powders and paprika together, then add water and Bragg Liquid Aminos.

2 Add the sweetcorn and blend until you have a creamy batter. Add some water to the batter if it is too thick, though you do need a fairly thick consistency.

3 Coat just one side of the spinach leaves with the batter. Don't coat both sides as they will stick to the tray. Place in a dehydrator tray, with the coated side up to avoid sticking. Dry till crisp.

WHAT YOU NEED

— 120 g baby spinach leaves
— 350 g sweetcorn
— 60 ml water
— 1 tsp Bragg Liquid Aminos
— 1 tsp paprika
— 1 tsp onion powder
— ½ tsp garlic powder

The simple combination of spinach, onion and sweetcorn is fantastic. These are an ideal complement for dips when enjoying a night in front of the telly.

SALT & PEPPER CRISPS

IMMUNE BOOSTER

Courgettes grow in abundance in the summer months. Use the larger ones because they shrink when dehydrated. I like to use a mandolin to slice these crisps as it's quick and the crisps turn out nice and even, but a sharp knife works just as well. Cayenne pepper is a great digestive aid that stimulates the flow of enzyme production and gastric juices.

WHAT YOU NEED

— 1 large courgette
— 4 tsp Udo's oil
— ¼ tsp celery salt
— ¼ tsp cayenne pepper
— ¼ tsp smoked paprika

The smoked paprika and cayenne add a nice bit of colour. Serve them with hummus, pesto or tapenade.

WHAT YOU DO

1 Slice the courgette into circles with the mandolin or knife.

2 Pour the Udo's oil into a bowl and add the celery salt, cayenne pepper and smoked paprika.

3 Coat the courgette rounds by rubbing them together with another slice to spread the oil around.

4 Place on a dehydrator tray and dry till crisp.

SWEET & TANGY LEFTOVERS

HEALTH ENHANCER

Sometimes you have shrivelled-up leftover apples that you don't want to throw away, especially if they are organic. This is a great way to use those leftovers from the fruit bowl. I slice apples, bananas, mango, pineapple, dip them in lemon juice to stop discoloration, and pop them on the dehydrator. Drying concentrates the fruit's sweetness, and the sweet slices are tinged with just the slightest bit of tartness from the lemon; a delicious combination.

WHAT YOU DO

1 You can use a mandolin to slice the apples, but mind your fingers. Alternatively, just use a sharp knife.

2 Core the apples, but don't waste the seeds. Apple seeds can be added to juice as they contain nitriloside compounds that protect us against disease.

3 Dip the apple slices in the lemon juice and place the slices on the dehydrator.

4 Dry until they have a consistency somewhere between chewy and crunchy.

WHAT YOU NEED

— *3 apples or other leftover fruits*
— *Juice of 1 lemon*

They are great for kids' lunchboxes, but don't let them get hooked as they are still full of sugars.

SWEET POTATO CRISPS

IMMUNE BOOSTER

If you are a crisp addict and are particularly partial to the salty flavour, this is a wonderful alternative. I use salted vegan bouillon for this recipe, which gives the crisps an authentic flavour. You can use a reduced salt bouillon if you prefer. Sweet potato crisps are delicious served with some pesto, hummus or tapenade. They have a low glycaemic load, are rich in vitamin A, and also provide fibre and vitamin C.

WHAT YOU NEED

— *2 sweet potatoes*
— *3 tbsp salted vegetable bouillon*
— *200 ml hot water*

If you continually graze and snack but want something healthy, these nibbles will rival your favourite fried crisps.

WHAT YOU DO

1 Wash and slice the sweet potatoes thinly, with the skin on.
2 Blend the vegetable bouillon with the hot water.
3 Coat the sliced sweet potatoes in the bouillon.
4 Place the sweet potatoes on the dehydrator until crisp.

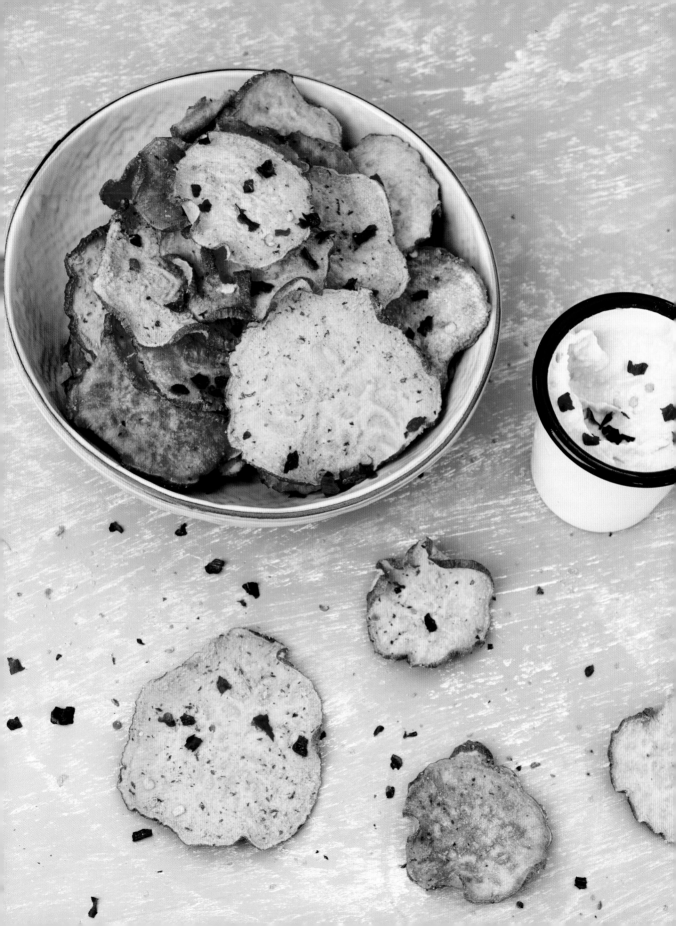

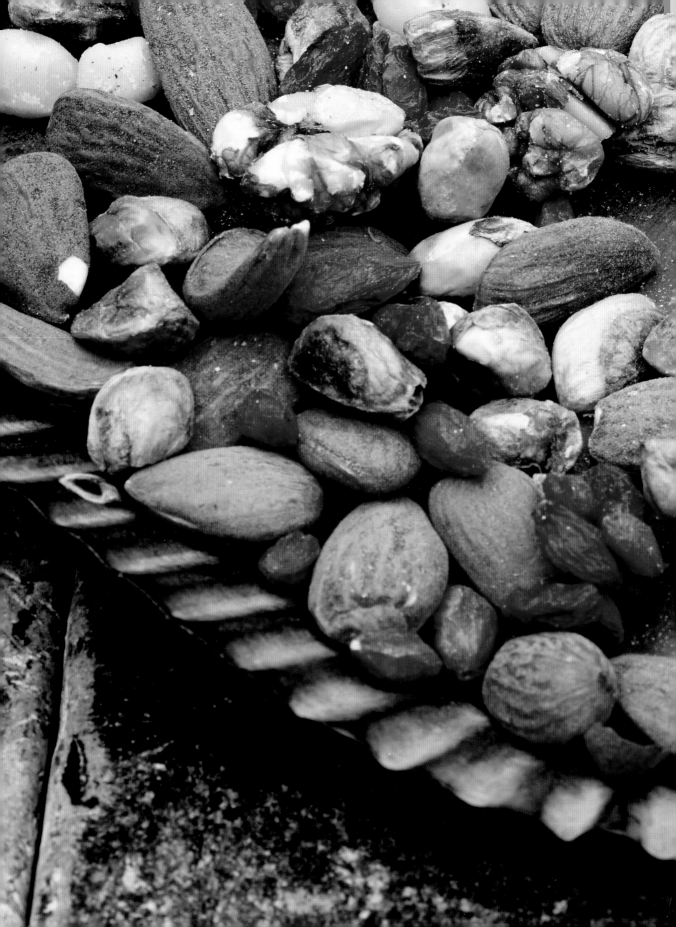

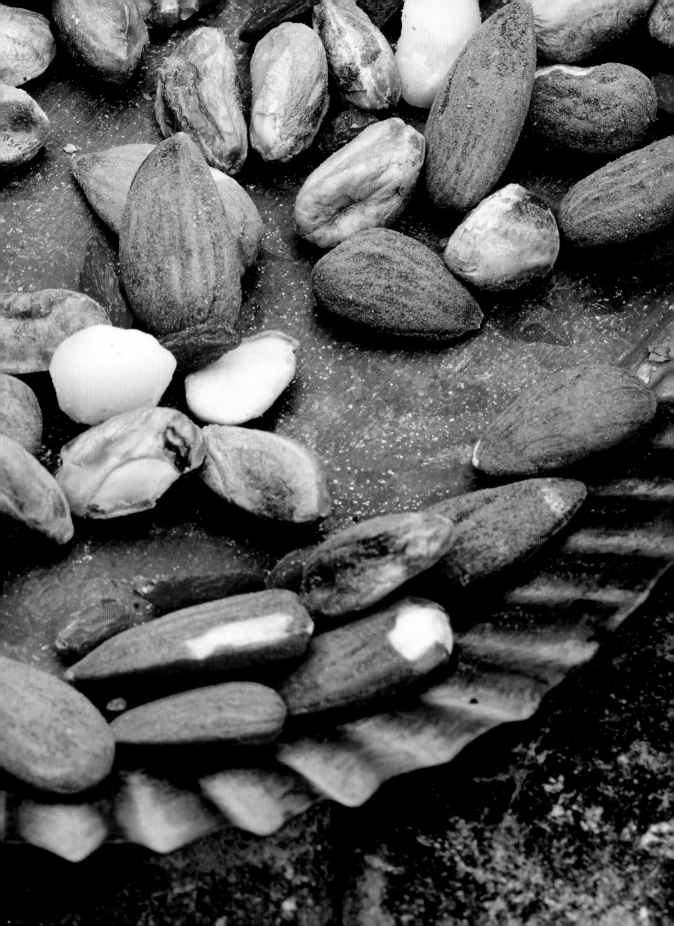

'Life is like an ice
cream cone, you
have to lick it one
day at a time.'
CHARLES M. SCHULZ

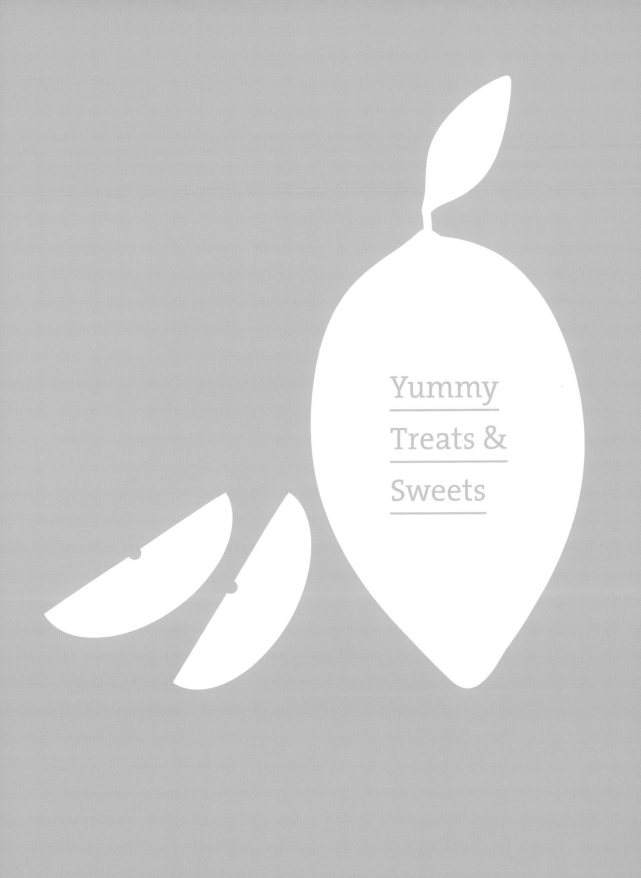

Yummy

Treats &

Sweets

If you want to give up sugar, cut calories or shed some extra pounds, there are many benefits to giving up the sugar habit. More often than not, losing weight is the main reason that people want to decrease the amount of sugar they consume. While this is a very good incentive, and will reduce the calorie disadvantage of those indulgent sweet treats, I am a realist and understand it may be hard to resist. I also know that if you ban them it makes them more appealing. So before we get to the goodies, let me outline the dangers and downsides those sweet temptations can have on your health. I know it sucks hearing that those sweet treats you love are bad for you, but I am doing my best to get you healthy.

Cholesterol is a problem caused by sugar and sugar derivatives such as high-fructose corn syrup. It's no secret that there are hidden sugars in vast amounts of commonly eaten foods ranging from fruit juices, probiotic drinks, sauces, salad dressings, cheese spreads and pretty much every processed food – even infant formulae. Remember, all those hidden sugars add up. Sugar can increase LDL cholesterol (bad cholesterol), which is a risk factor for cardiovascular disease. As we all know it's addictive; the more sugars that are added to your food, the more of it you will want. Food companies count on you developing an addictive relationship with their foods. Don't be duped, read the label – or better still, make your own treats.

Cancer cells thrive on sugar; they have many more receptor cells for capturing sugar than healthy cells. The molecular biology of cancer cells requires more glucose to feed them. For some people, cancer cells grow faster and stronger when the person's sugar levels are frequently above normal. Cutting down our intake of sugar cuts off an important food supply to cancer cells. It's not just people who are diagnosed with cancer whom this affects. Each of us generates new cancer cells each day in our bodies. A healthy immune system deals with these so that they don't become an issue, but how can you build a strong immune system with foods that increase your risk of cancer?

Sugar:

- elevates LDL cholesterol;
- disturbs brain chemistry;
- increases weight and obesity;
- raises blood sugar levels;
- increases risk factor for kidney disease and diabetes;
- feeds fungus, yeasts and bacteria; and
- rots teeth.

When you learn about the dangers that eating certain foods can cause, and how those foods can escalate health problems, you want to do what you can to avoid them.

What to do about sugar

When you eat sugar, whether it's white table sugar, agave nectar, honey, corn syrup, saccharine, aspartame, xylitol or fruit sugar (fructose), you get an instant spike in the glucose level of the blood. Sugars are like a time bomb ticking within our systems because your pancreas must secrete large amounts of insulin to stop blood sugar levels from rising too high. Every time you eat sugary foods, they cause an imbalance in your body chemistry. The extra insulin pushes your system into overload, which tends to make the blood sugar levels fall to levels that are too low. Even the so-called 'healthy sugar alternatives' can actually increase your cravings for sugar, which is all bad news for your health and your waistline.

Many health advocates recommend agave syrup, or agave nectar, as a healthy alternative to sugar. While this sounds healthy, they don't inform you that it's processed, high in fructose, is absorbed as sugar by the body and causes unwanted weight gain. I am very sceptical of alternative sweeteners that are promoted as health foods because they usually promote some kind of fad that can be damaging in the long term.

Use stevia to sweeten and reduce your sugar intake. Stevia comes from a plant and has a low glycaemic load, so it won't spike your blood sugars; in fact,it actually helps to regulate blood-sugar levels. It can be bought in liquid or powder form. The sachets are very handy, but the drops work well in juices and sauces as they dissolve easily. Stevia is about 400 times sweeter than sugar: ½ teaspoon of stevia is equal to one cup of sugar. It has been used in Japan for years to replace sugar, and the Japanese consume over 300,000 pounds of it each year. Stevia has become widely available as a sweetener since its approval for use by the EU in 2011. It will help you to avoid the treats and sweets aisles, and get you over the hump of giving up the demon sugar.

Treats are meant for special occasions, which should be celebrated – I am not a total spoilsport! – but they are not for every day. Much as we like to think we deserve a treat each day or need a reward, treats and sweets are not required foods for your body. You will notice that all the treats and sweets are 'health enhancer' recipes. Fruits and dried fruits are often used to sweeten treats and sweets, but they still contain sugars and as such they should be used sparingly. In other words, don't scoff the whole batch of cookies yourself. Nudge, nudge, wink, wink! Seriously, once you find a healthy replacement for your usual treat you won't be inclined to surrender to the melt-in-the-mouth products any more.

It may take some time because sugar has such a strong hold on us and is so addictive. Be prepared for those cravings; try the Divine & Decadent Tiramisu, the Guilt-free Cookies or Berry N-ice Cream. Or, if you are Nuts About Ice Cream, make your own ice cream at home – you don't even need an expensive ice cream maker. Have a weekend treat that will help you break the dependence on sugar and phase out those store-bought treats. If you want to be healthier, happier and thinner, cutting back on sugar will definitely be good for your figure and amazing for your health. Stay strong!

NUTS ABOUT ICE CREAM

HEALTH ENHANCER

This ice cream is a treat on Saturday evenings for the guests at the Hippocrates Health Institute. Their talented executive chef Ken Blue is very strict about sugars, because every time you eat refined sugary foods, they cause an imbalance in your body chemistry. He uses maple flavour in this ice cream, not maple syrup; I thought it would be difficult to find, but I had no trouble sourcing it online. If you don't have it, that's okay as the ice cream works well without it. Use the nut milk from page 59 or, alternatively, you can use a carton of almond milk for convenience. You can halve the quantity if you want a smaller batch, but when you divvy it out, it will disappear quickly.

WHAT YOU DO

1 If you don't have an ice cream maker, place all ingredients except for the walnuts in a food processor. Process until creamy.

2 Chop the walnuts roughly and stir into the mix.

3 Place in an air-tight container and chill in the freezer for a few hours till the ice cream hardens.

4 Let it sit for about 15 minutes or so to soften before scooping into serving bowls.

WHAT YOU NEED

— 50 g walnuts
— 1 litre nut milk
— 30 ml vanilla extract
— 1 tbsp cinnamon
— 15 ml maple flavour
— 5 drops stevia

I like to add a few walnuts to give it a crunchy nutty texture. You will be nuts about this one!

DIVINE & DECADENT TIRAMISU

HEALTH ENHANCER

I tinkered about with various coffee substitutes to give this dessert an authentic flavour. There are a few really good caffeine-free coffees, they come in different flavours – java, rich roast, almond, amaretto – and really taste good. I use Teeccino, a herbal coffee made with barley, chicory root, figs, almonds and roasted carob. You will find it in good health food shops or on the internet.

A love affair with coffee can easily spiral. There is no doubt that coffee gives you a lift. However, that temporary increase in energy you experience is short-lived and before you know it, you're having three or four cups a day just to keep yourself ticking over. Try this for birthday treats or dinner parties – the cream filling is silky and rich, with a divine coffee flavour.

WHAT YOU NEED FOR CAKE BASE

— 220 g pecans
— 150 g dates
— 1 tsp carob powder
— 3 tsp rich roast Teeccino
— 1 tsp vanilla extract
— 1 tsp shredded coconut

WHAT YOU NEED FOR CREAM FILLING

— 280 g macadamia nuts
— 250 ml water
— 1 banana
— 2 tbsp coconut oil
— 1 tbsp nutritional yeast (optional)
— 1 tsp vanilla extract

This divine and decadent tiramisu is rich, luscious and almost sinfully good.

WHAT YOU DO FOR CAKE BASE

1 Soak the nuts and dates overnight in water.
2 Drain off water from nuts and dates and process in a blender. Add the remaining ingredients and blend until the mix holds together.
3 Use a springform pan to make it easy to remove the cake from the pan. Another tip is to sprinkle a dusting of coconut flakes on the base to stop the crust from sticking to the bottom of the pan.
4 Press the mix into the pan to form the crust.

WHAT YOU DO FOR CREAM FILLING

5 Throw all the ingredients into your blender and blend to a creamy consistency.
6 Pour the cream mixture over the crust in the springform pan and smooth right up to edge of the pan.
7 Pop the cake into the freezer for about 3 hours. Allow to thaw before slicing.
8 Sprinkle with a little carob powder before serving.

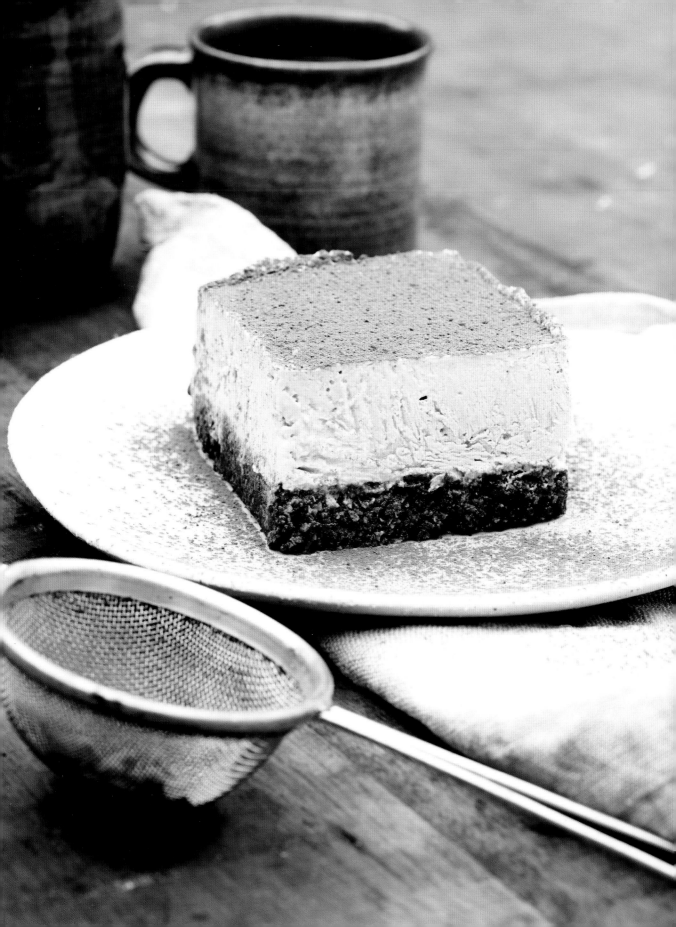

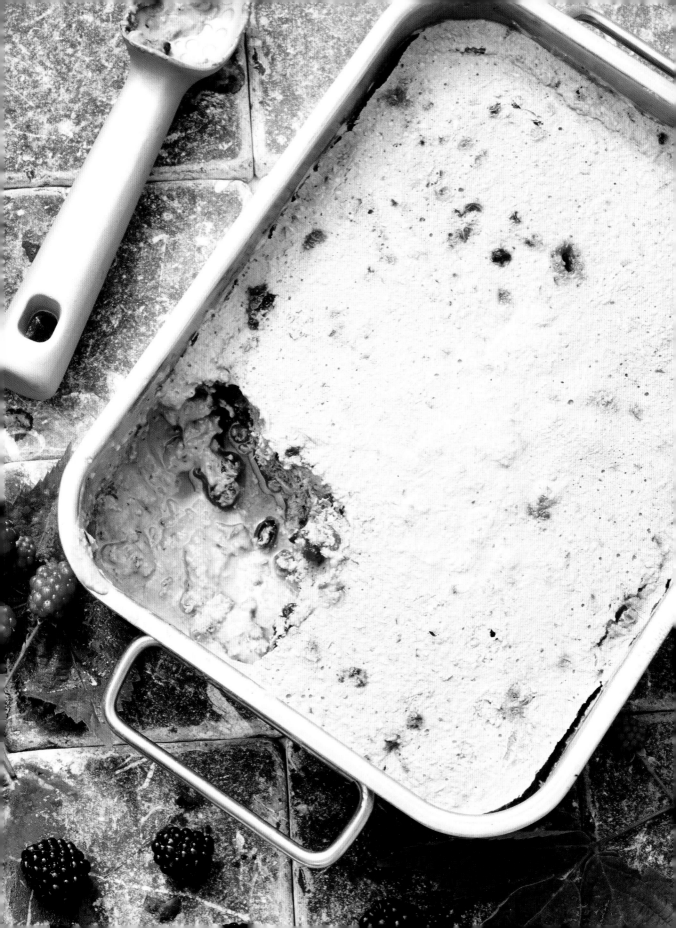

BERRY N-ICE CREAM

HEALTH ENHANCER

This delicious ice cream is beyond easy. Keep a few bananas in the freezer so you can whip this up in a flash.

Strawberries, raspberries, blueberries, blackberries and cranberries are rich in polyphenols, a compound found in foods that are purple or red in colour and which protects your body from cell damage. The berries in this recipe add some super nutrients, so you won't feel like you've fallen off the healthy-eating wagon. You can use the blank screen that is provided with your juicer, or use a food processor to blend the fruit. If you want to make the ice cream into swirls, you can buy an extra attachment, but you can just use a scoop or spoon instead. Oh, and don't forget to lick the spoon!

WHAT YOU DO

1 Peel the bananas and freeze overnight.
2 Mix the berries, vanilla and stevia together and process with the peeled bananas.
3 If you like a soft ice cream, add 125 ml of nut milk. Enjoy!

WHAT YOU NEED

— *2 bananas*
— *300 g mixed berries*
— *3 drops vanilla essence*
— *3 drops liquid stevia (optional)*
— *nut milk (optional)*

I like to add some vanilla essence for a richer flavour. Try and source a non-alcoholic brand – most health stores carry them.

LEMON MERINGUE PIE

HEALTH ENHANCER

The classic version of lemon meringue pie is made with egg yolks and sweetened condensed milk, which are all ingredients we want to avoid. This lighter version will excite your palate and won't leave you feeling bloated. It's not a true meringue, as there are no eggs in this recipe, but it tastes delicious. If you always share dessert, this is one that you may actually fight over.

WHAT YOU NEED FOR CRUST

— 160 g pecans, soaked
— 70 g raisins, soaked in lemon juice
— 1 lemon
— 20 g desiccated coconut

WHAT YOU NEED FOR LEMON PIE FILLING

— 250 ml almond nut milk
— 230 g coconut oil, softened
— 2 tbsp lecithin powder
— Juice of 3 lemons
— 4 tsp alcohol-free vanilla extract
— 3 drops liquid stevia

WHAT YOU NEED FOR MERINGUE TOPPING

— 190 ml almond nut milk
— 140 g macadamia nuts
— 1 tsp lemon juice
— 1 tsp alcohol-free vanilla extract
— 3 drops liquid stevia
— 1 tsp lecithin powder
— 60 g coconut oil, softened

WHAT YOU DO FOR CRUST

1 Soak the nuts overnight in water.
2 Soak the raisins in the juice of a lemon.
3 Drain the nuts and raisins and process in a blender.
4 Then press the nut and raisin mix into a pie tin to form the crust. Use a spring-form tin to make it easy to remove the pie from the tin. Another tip is to sprinkle some coconut flakes on the base of the tin to stop the crust from sticking to the bottom.

WHAT YOU DO FOR LEMON FILLING

1 Blend all the ingredients except lecithin powder and coconut oil.
2 Blend the oil and lecithin powder on low to a creamy consistency.
3 Pour mixture over crust and smooth right up to edge of the pie dish.
4 Pop the pie into the freezer for about 3 hours.
5 Remove and keep in fridge till ready to eat.

WHAT YOU DO FOR MERINGUE TOPPING

1 Blend all ingredients together and place a dollop of the cream over the pie just before serving.
2 Decorate with a few slices of lemon or mint.

Sensational layers of creamy citrus filling finished with luscious cream topping.

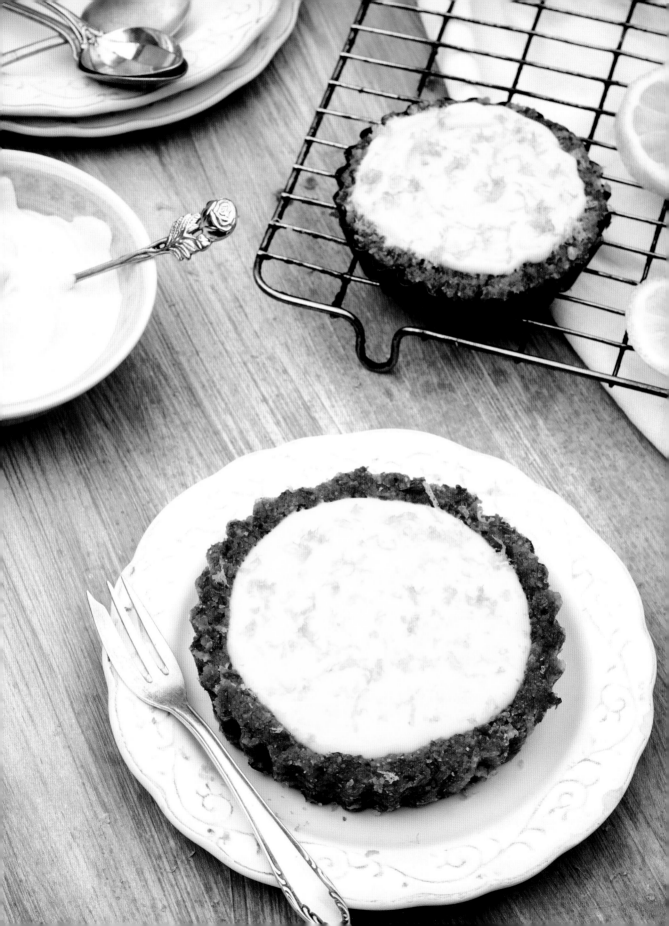

DAIRY-FREE CRÈME CHANTILLY

This famous whipped cream from the medieval French market town is a perfect topping for desserts, but it is usually made with heavy cream and sweetened with sugar.

Basically, the human body does not require milk after weaning, and by that stage, we produce less of the lactase enzymes necessary for its digestion. Lactose is made from one molecule of glucose and one molecule of galactose. It is a disaccharide, a type of sugar that must be broken down in the small intestine by lactase enzymes. If it is not properly absorbed, it ferments in the digestive system and is the cause of many digestive problems.

WHAT YOU NEED

— 190 ml almond milk
— 140 g macadamia nuts
— 1 tsp lemon juice
— 1 tsp alcohol-free vanilla extract
— 3 drops stevia
— 1 tsp lecithin powder
— 60 g coconut oil, softened

WHAT YOU DO

1   Blend all ingredients together and top dessert just before serving.

Infused with vanilla extract, this Dairy-free Crème Chantilly is simple but decadent.

ENERGY BARS

Better energy levels are a result of eating better food, and these delicious energy bars will keep you going throughout the day. I like to use almonds as they have a nice rich flavour, and I also add some millet because it is a non-acid-forming grain and contains a myriad of beneficial nutrients. Millet is readily available, and is one of the least allergenic and most digestible gluten-free grains. You can, of course, omit it if you don't have it to hand.

WHAT YOU DO

1   Soak the nuts and millet overnight in water and drain. Also soak the dates overnight in the juice of the orange. Save the rind. The dates will absorb most of the juice.

2   Chop the rind of the orange finely in your food processor, then simply push the nuts, dates and rind through your juicer using the blank screen.

3   Turn the mixture onto parchment paper, cover with another sheet of paper and roll with a rolling pin.

4   Form into bars and place in the dehydrator overnight. Enjoy!

WHAT YOU NEED

— *600 g almonds, soaked overnight*
— *460 g dates, soaked overnight in the juice of 1 orange*
— *2 tbsp millet, soaked overnight*
— *1 orange*

My girls like a crunchier texture, so I dehydrate these bars overnight.

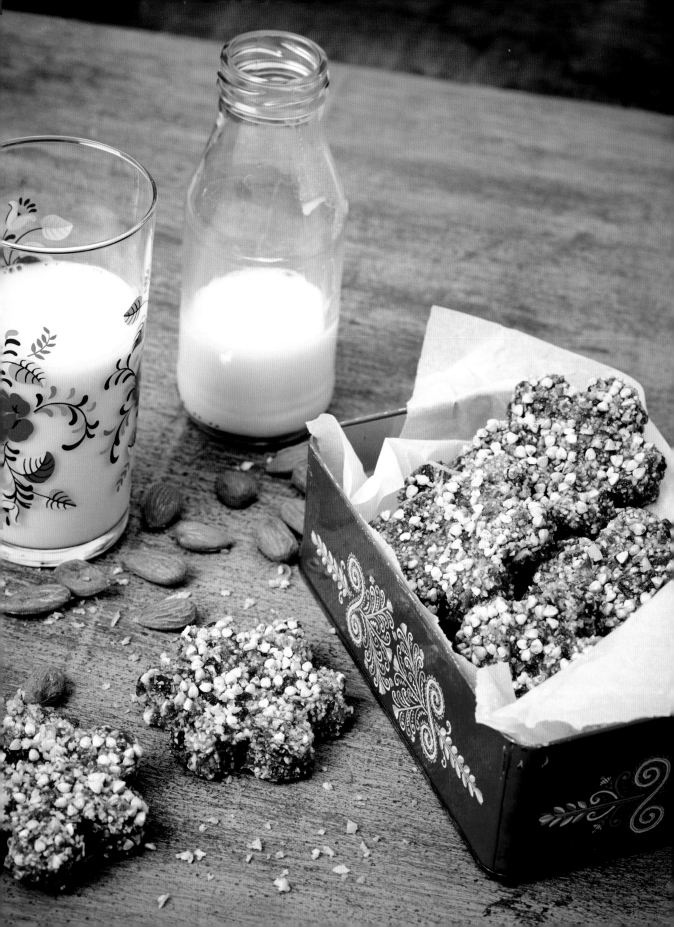

GUILT-FREE COOKIES

HEALTH ENHANCER

A super healthy option for a sweet tooth, these guilt-free cookies are better than the usual sugar bomb you get from store-bought cookies. Another bonus for those who have to worry about gluten, these cookies are gluten-free. The sweet ripe bananas with the coconut and touch of vanilla are a delicious combination. Besides being delicious, you can savour these cookies without regret. You simply cannot go wrong with them; they come out perfectly every time.

WHAT YOU DO

1 Mix all ingredients together until they are well combined, and refrigerate for half an hour.

2 Scoop into small balls, roll in your hands and flatten with your palm, or cut with a cookie-cutter.

3 Place in the dehydrator and dry overnight until the cookies are crisp to the touch on the outside and soft in the centre.

WHAT YOU NEED

— *2 ripe bananas, mashed*
— *50 g shredded coconut*
— *¼ cup coconut butter*
— *60 g chopped nuts*
— *1 tsp alcohol-free vanilla extract*
— *50 g dried buckwheat*
— *3 drops stevia (optional)*

Try these out on your friends who are partial to chomping on cookies. They won't believe they have NO added sugar. Does it get any better?

MAMMY'S HOME-MADE BREAD

HEALTH ENHANCER

My mum was a fabulous baker, and although I don't eat much bread these days, this fresh home-made bread is still a favourite with the family. I have deviated a little from my mother's trusted recipe by making this bread with rice milk and spelt flour. While I can almost hear her say, 'Don't fix what is not broken', spelt is much easier to digest than wheat. It has a nutty and slightly sweet flavour. I love to add nutritious seeds into the mix, as they give this bread a nice crunchy texture.

WHAT YOU NEED

— *340 g brown spelt flour*
— *300 ml organic rice milk*
— *1 tbsp sesame seeds*
— *4 tbsp pumpkin seeds*
— *3 tsp gluten-free baking powder*
— *Juice of ½ a lemon*
— *Knob coconut butter*

I have been more specific about the amounts here, as when baking bread it's important to have the quantities correct.

WHAT YOU DO

1   Preheat the oven to gas mark 4/175°C.
2   Mix all the dry ingredients together, sieving the baking powder into the dry mix.
3   Add the rice milk and lemon juice and mix thoroughly until a thick dough forms.
4   Lightly coat a 450 g loaf tin with the coconut butter.
5   Pour the mixture into the tin until it's about three-quarters full.
6   Bake for 45 minutes to an hour.
7   Turn out onto a baking tray and check to see if the base of the loaf is firm.

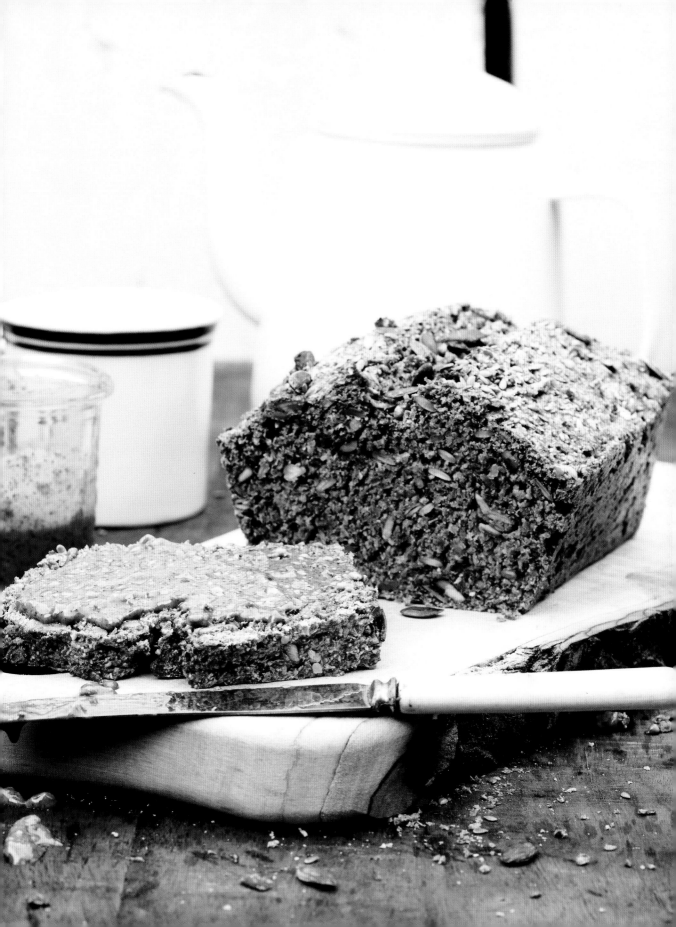

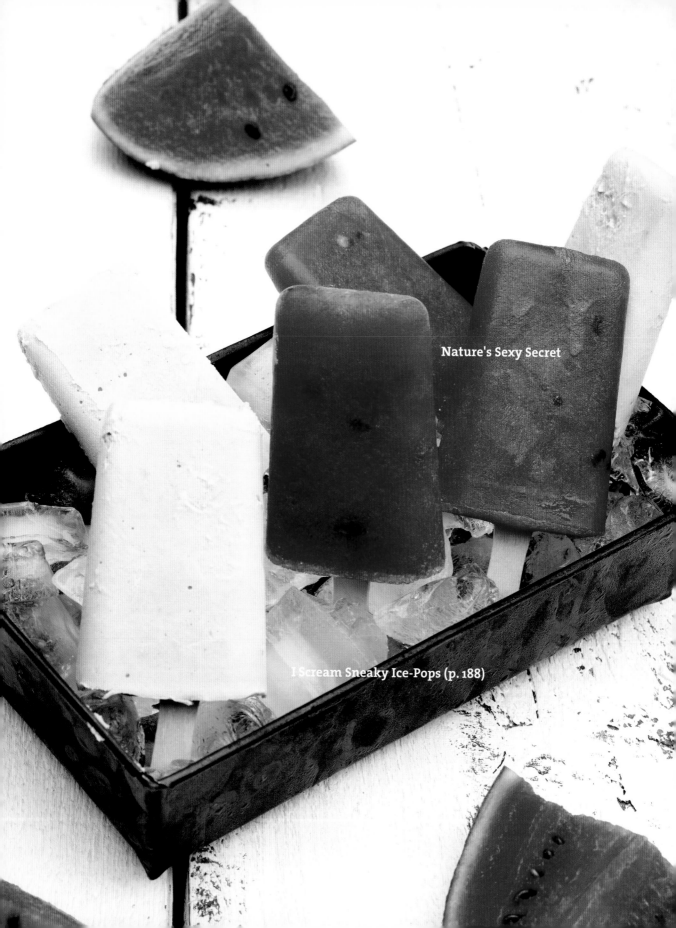

Nature's Sexy Secret

I Scream Sneaky Ice-Pops (p. 188)

NATURE'S SEXY SECRET

HEALTH ENHANCER

Who would have guessed that one of the summer's greatest and most refreshing pleasures, watermelon, is great for your libido? The secret lies in the rind; this contains a nutrient known as citrulline, which is converted into arginine in the body. Arginine boosts nitric oxide, which relaxes blood vessels. I know it sounds complicated, but isn't it interesting how Mother Nature has all the tricks to turn you on and get you in the right mood? These ice lollies will easily woo anyone who tries them.

WHAT YOU DO

1 Remove the skin from the watermelon and process with the lime juice.

2 Pour into moulds and stick them in the freezer till the right moment and enjoy nature's not-so-guilty secret. Let the wooing begin.

WHAT YOU NEED

— *1 watermelon*
— *Juice of 1 lime*
— *Ice lolly moulds*

Juice the rind to get all that sensual goodness. I also use the seeds as they are rich in proteins and B vitamins and minerals. They look pretty in the lollies, too, but you can take them out before blending if you prefer.

WALNUT BONBONS

HEALTH ENHANCER

These bonbons can be made in batches and stored in the fridge. If you are wary of trying to give up sugar because of previous broken commitments, why not try these bonbons? They will help pacify your sweet tooth. I'm not suggesting you won't miss your favourite choccie bar, but learning how sugar affects you can reduce your susceptibility to those sweet pleasures. The great thing is that they're ready in about 10 minutes. They remind me of marzipan.

WHAT YOU NEED

— *50 g crunchy hazelnut butter*
— *1 tsp alcohol-free vanilla extract*
— *140 g walnuts, chopped*
— *80 g dates*

I like to use my juicer for bonbons as it brings the mixture together nice and tight, but you can use a food processor.

WHAT YOU DO

1 Using the blank screen from your juicer (or a food processor), process half of the walnuts, all of the dates and the vanilla extract till fully combined.

2 Blend in the hazelnut butter.

3 Roll into balls, pressing the mixture together firmly so it will hold.

4 Chop the remaining walnuts finely and roll the bonbons in the chopped nuts.

5 Place the bonbons onto parchment paper and pop in the fridge for 10 minutes.

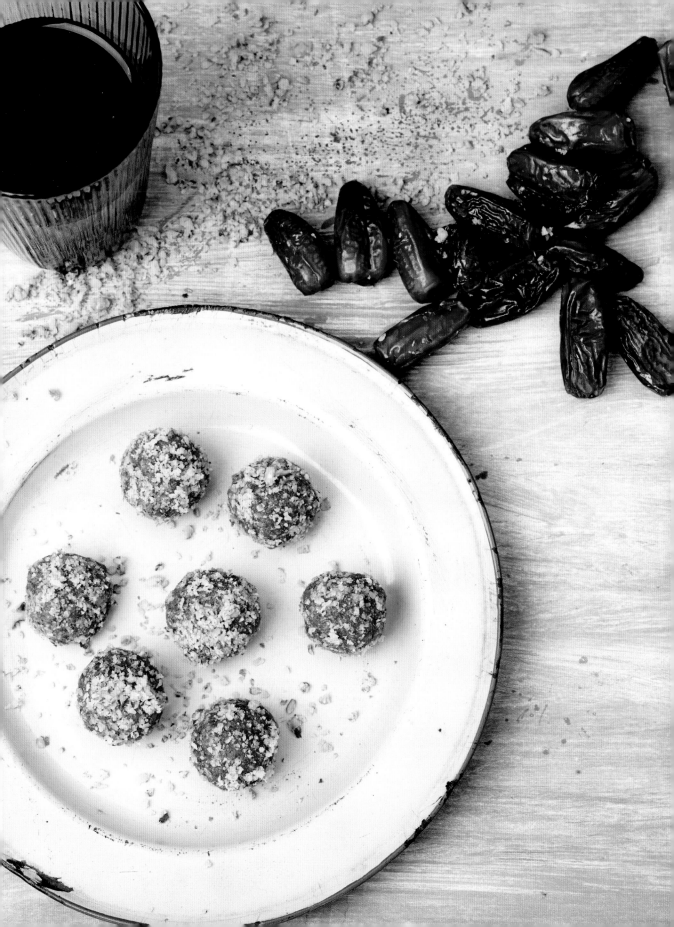

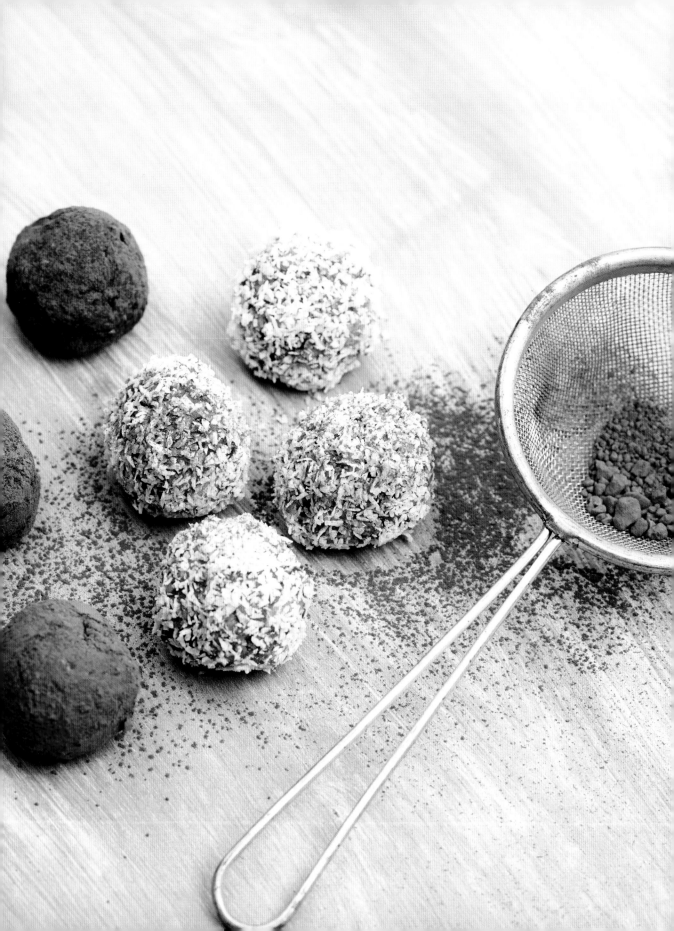

SWEET INDULGENCE

HEALTH ENHANCER

Save these truffles for those moments when you need an extra bit of TLC; they are the perfect antidote to the sugar blues.

These are an indulgent treat that has a lovely citrus flavour, smothered in shredded coconut. The skin of citrus fruit is actually the most beneficial part as it contains the most vitamin C and bioflavonoids.

This is probably the easiest recipe for truffles around. They are so simple – you just mix the ingredients together. I use the blank screen that comes with the juicer, as it creates a tighter mixture that sticks together well.

WHAT YOU DO

1 Soak the nuts and seeds for 15 minutes and rinse.
2 Grate the rind of the orange in a processor.
3 Add all ingredients except the shredded coconut to your juicer through the blank screen, or use a blender.
4 Roll the mix into balls and coat each ball in shredded coconut.
5 Refrigerate for 20 minutes – and try not to indulge too much!

WHAT YOU NEED

— *200 g pecan nuts, soaked and rinsed*
— *1 tsp sesame seeds, soaked and rinsed*
— *150 g dates, soaked in orange juice*
— *50 g shredded coconut*
— *Juice and rind of 1 orange*

Although these truffles are quite luscious, you won't feel heavy after eating them.

LOTS OF LOVELY HEARTS

It's easy to win hearts with these lovely sweets. Sometimes the simplest of ingredients create the most delectable taste experiences. With just a few simple ingredients, you can produce these love-infused beauties. They are irresistible, so before you submit to an impulse to buy sweets at the checkout counter, make a batch. I use strawberries for the pink ones, and a little turmeric to make the yellow ones.

WHAT YOU NEED

— *1 ripe banana*
— *400 ml tin coconut milk*
— *4 dates, soaked in lemon juice*
— *150 g strawberries*
— *Pinch turmeric*
— *Heart-shaped moulds*

WHAT YOU DO

1 Process banana and coconut milk together.
2 Add strawberries to half the mixture, and turmeric to the other half.
3 Pour into heart-shaped moulds and freeze.
4 Thaw before demolishing the lot.

Be warned ... one just won't be enough, but if you share, you may make your way into someone's heart!

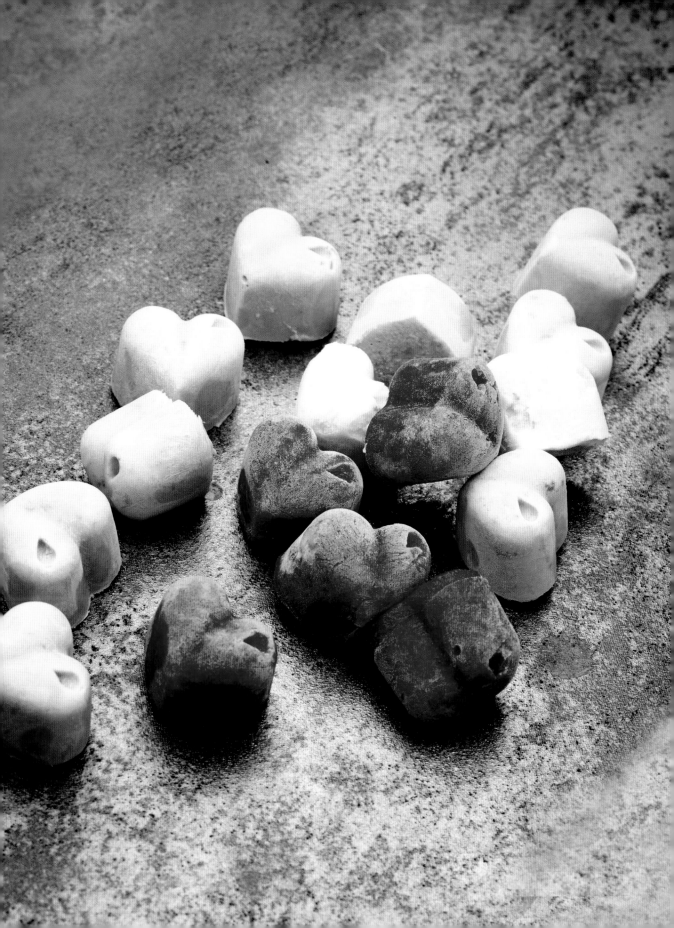

NO-SUGAR, NO-CHEESE-CAKE

HEALTH ENHANCER

This recipe is one I am really eager to share with you: first, there is not a bit of cheese in sight and second, there is no refined sugar in this recipe. The decorating for this recipe was inspired by Kristina Carrillo-Bucaram, a pioneer in the local, organic food co-operative movement. The strawberries are used to layer in between the mixture, and are the crowning glory of this No-sugar, No-cheese-cake. Go on, show your guests just how amazing you are.

WHAT YOU NEED FOR CRUST

— *160 g walnuts*
— *160 g pecans*
— *150 g dates*
— *1 tsp alcohol-free vanilla extract*
— *2 tbsp coconut oil*

WHAT YOU NEED FOR FILLING

— *900 g strawberries (180 g for blending, the rest sliced for layers)*
— *2 frozen bananas*
— *800 ml tinned coconut milk*
— *140 g macadamia nuts*
— *1 tbsp alcohol-free vanilla extract*
— *3 drops stevia*

WHAT YOU NEED FOR STRAWBERRY GLAZE

— *160 g frozen strawberries*
— *80 g dates*

The secret with this cake is not to have too many slices. I guarantee you will be tempted.

WHAT TO DO FOR CRUST

1 Soak the nuts and dates overnight.
2 Drain off water from nuts and dates and process with the vanilla in a blender. Gradually add the coconut oil till the crust holds together.
3 Use a springform pan to make it easy to remove the cake from the pan. Another tip is to sprinkle a dust of coconut flakes on the base of the pan to stop the crust from sticking.
4 Press the mix into the pan to form the crust.

WHAT YOU DO FOR FILLING

1 Throw all the ingredients (except the reserved sliced strawberries) into your blender and blend to a creamy consistency. If the mixture is too thick, add a little extra coconut oil to enable blending.
2 Slice the strawberries and layer on top of crust.
3 Pour half the cream mixture over the strawberries and smooth right up to the edge of the tin.
4 Add a second layer of sliced strawberries. Add the remaining cream mixture.

WHAT YOU DO FOR STRAWBERRY GLAZE

1 Blend the berries and dates in your blender till nice and smooth.
2 Pour on top of your cake, and top with sliced strawberries.
3 Pop the cake into the freezer for about 3 hours.

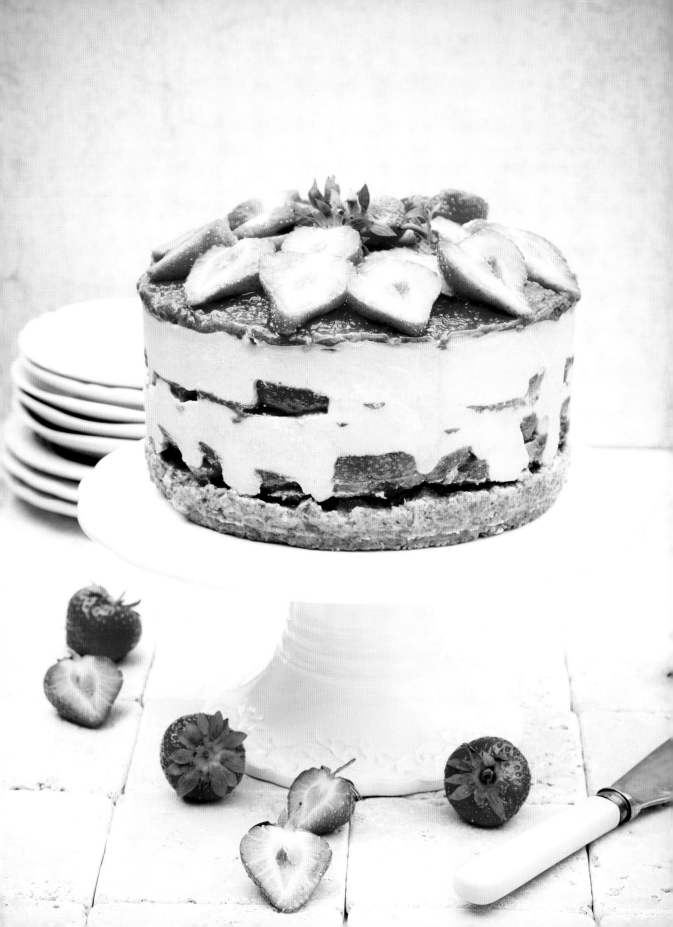

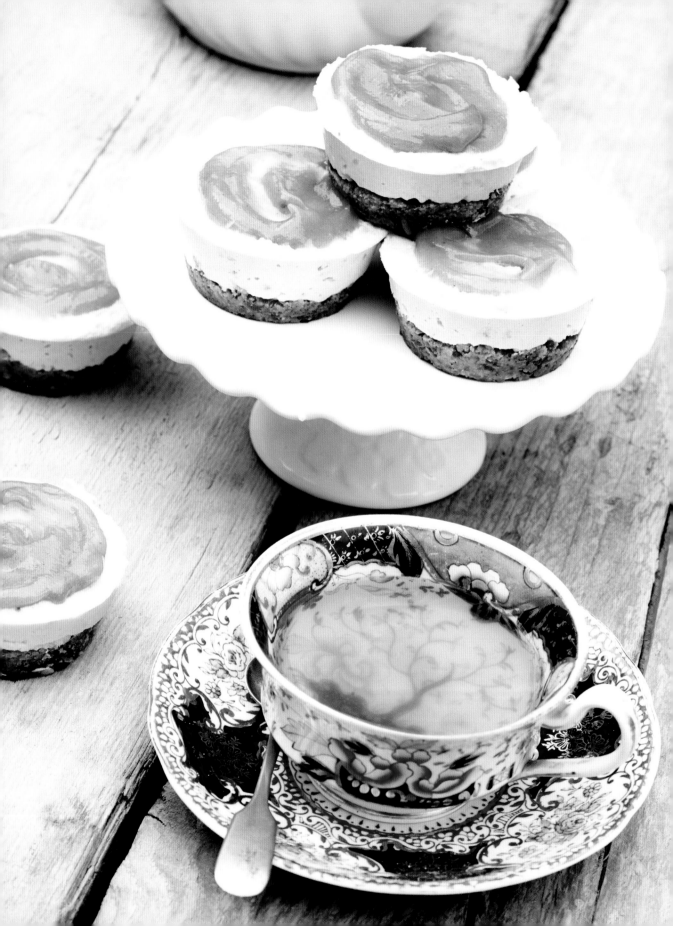

NOT-SO-NAUGHTY BUT NICE PIES

HEALTH ENHANCER

These pies sound a bit naughty but are, in fact, full of good fats. I think everyone loves sweet pie, but most of them are so heavy they would sink a ship. Pecans have a sweetness that works beautifully in desserts. Soak the dates in orange juice to soften them, as it gives a lovely flavour to the base and fudge topping. Dates have a high amount of natural sugars that definitely score high on the naughty list.

WHAT YOU DO FOR CRUST

1. Drain juice off dates. Pulse the walnuts and pecans together in a food processor.
2. Add dates and process until it forms a sticky dough.
3. Press the mixture into a small pie moulds and press tightly.
4. Store in the fridge while you make the cream layer.

WHAT YOU DO FOR CREAM FILLING

1. Blend the bananas, coconut milk, dates and vanilla extract together.
2. Pour over pie crust.

WHAT YOU DO FOR FUDGE TOPPING

1. Combine dates, water and vanilla extract together till you have a nice, sticky fudge consistency.
2. Spoon over pies before serving.

WHAT YOU NEED FOR CRUST

— 160 g walnuts
— 160 g pecans
— 150 g dates, soaked in orange juice
— 1 orange

WHAT YOU NEED FOR CREAM FILLING

— 2 frozen bananas
— 400 ml tin coconut milk
— 4 dates, soaked in lemon juice
— ½ tsp alcohol-free vanilla extract

WHAT YOU NEED FOR FUDGE TOPPING

— 150 g dates
— 60 ml water
— ½ tsp alcohol-free vanilla extract

Topped with a rich fudge, these pies are mouth-watering.

I SCREAM SNEAKY ICE-POPS

HEALTH ENHANCER

With no artificial colourings or flavourings, these scrumptious, creamy ice-pops are so much nicer than the commercially made ones. They are a perfect treat if the kids are screaming for something to eat. Big and little kids will love them. I add a little turmeric to give the ice-pops their yummy yellow colour. Turmeric has powerful healing properties, which is why I like to sneak it into as many foods as I can, even ice pops.

The thing about these ice pops is that they are so damn good, you may not want to share them.

WHAT YOU NEED

— *1 ripe banana*
— *400 ml tin coconut milk*
— *4 dates, soaked in lemon juice*
— *Pinch of turmeric*

WHAT YOU DO

1 Pit and soak the dates in lemon juice till soft.
2 Blend all ingredients until smooth.
3 Pour into ice pop moulds and freeze.

Simple, and as the name suggests, a little sneaky.

THE SWEETEST THING SYRUP

There are few things in life as simple as this sweet syrup. It's a divine addition to everything from granola bars to dessert toppings and sweet pie crusts. Dates are natural sweeteners, but don't overdo it; they should be eaten in moderation.

While I prefer to use dates, if you are not a date lover, it can be made successfully with raisins. Lemon juice helps to keep the syrup fresh – it will keep for a week in the fridge.

WHAT YOU DO

1 Blend the ingredients through your juicer or use a blender until you have a smooth consistency.

WHAT YOU NEED

— *300 g Medjool dates, pitted*
— *1 tbsp lemon juice*
— *Cinnamon or vanilla essence, to taste*

An oh-soooo-good embellishment for all things sweet.

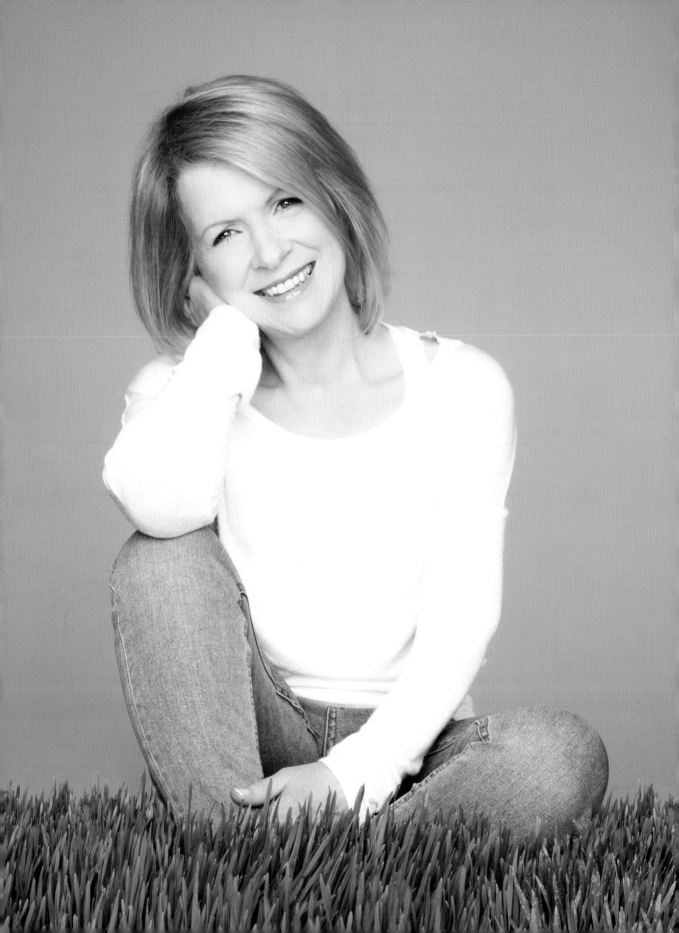

WHY
I TAKE
SUPPLEMENTS

You might wonder if you need to take supplements when you eat raw or living foods – or indeed any foods. There are a few reasons. Nowadays our soils are so depleted of minerals from intensive farming. Dr Linus Pauling, twice Nobel prize-winner, said, 'You can trace every sickness, every disease and every ailment to a mineral deficiency.' Many people are malnourished, despite the fact that they have what appears to be a reasonably healthy diet. Then they cook their foods and further deplete the foods of nutrients. Eating these foods can lead to a compromised immune system, which is a recipe for ill-health. As I want to optimise my health, I supplement daily with food-grade supplements.

The type of supplements you use is important, as many contain chemicals, preservatives, pesticides, sugars, fillers and gluten. There are many supplements on the market these days that have little effect, yet people spend a lot of their hard-earned cash on them. People take synthetic supplements without realising that they can do more harm than good. Watch out for supplements that contain synthesised additives to ensure that you are not ingesting chemical solvents that have harmful side effects that will weaken your immune system.

There is a vast difference between natural nutrients and synthetic nutrients. Your body cannot absorb synthetic man-made supplements. Your body simply is not designed to utilise them, in fact the body will try hard to excrete any synthetic substances you ingest. Natural nutrients, on the other hand, are readily absorbed by the body because we are biologically pro-grammed to absorb naturally occurring compounds as genuine nutrients.

There are many benefits to using natural supplements. Here are some of the ones I take regularly. I can't really list these in order of preference, as they all contain specific nutrients that I want to include in my diet.

Digestive Enzymes Despite the fact that I eat mostly enzyme-rich foods, I would not be without digestive enzymes because they provide essential nutrients, vitamins, minerals and enhance digestion of foods. They are also said to help increase the electromagnetic frequency around the cell and fight off free-radical damage, which is the cause of disease and aging. A lack of enzymes can lead to all sorts of problems: the overgrowth of parasites, food allergies, constipation, indigestion, gas and bloating.

Chlorella is one supplement I take regularly. It's an excellent source of protein that is easily digested. It's fabulous for sugar cravings as it balances blood sugars. It also detoxifies the body of heavy metals. If you have had procedures involving radiation, x-rays, travel on flights, sit in front of a computer, or have mercury fillings, chlorella is a good bet to stave off the ravages of modern life.

B 12 I believe is a must for everyone. It helps to increase the formation of haemoglobin (iron) levels in the blood. It also enhances energy production and endurance, and plays a key role in the normal functioning of the brain and nervous system.

Vitamin D Most of us don't get enough of this valuable vitamin, especially when we live in Northern climates. Vitamin D is essential for the absorption of calcium. The calcium in many synthetic supplements is secreted by the body because it cannot be absorbed. I use a naturally occurring source of vitamin D from shitake mushrooms and rice bran, because I know that good general health, bone health, a strong immune system and anti-cancer benefits have been directly connected to the intake of vitamin D.

Probiotics I take a good probiotic to provide healthy bacteria. We need good bacteria to populate the digestive tract to help with digestion, cell development and the strengthening of the immune system. Probiotics are especially helpful to replace beneficial bacteria destroyed by taking antibiotics.

Multivitamin My hubby and I also take a 100% pure, wholefood multivitamin, mineral and herb formula, created especially for women's and men's health. Women and men have very different needs, and many adult men and women are living with hormone imbalances, which can result in weight gain, fatigue, emotional imbalance and mood swings, decreased concentration, as well as loss of libido.

Enhanced Turmeric The potent plant compounds in turmeric are considered to make it the most powerful healing rhizome on the planet. Curcuminoids enhance brain function and offer anti-cancer effects, as well as helping to heal wounds, aid digestion, relieve pain and reduce inflammation. Since inflammation is responsible for playing a large role in many diseases, if you have arthritis, rheumatism, muscular problems or memory loss, you should add turmeric to your daily diet and ensure you are getting good quantities of it.

Research is underway to develop pharmaceutical drugs out of turmeric-based ingredients to fight disease. The biological activity of turmeric as a healing agent explains why companies are so interested in it and why they have filed so many patent applications for it. It can be taken in a supplement form, which is useful, because the enhanced supplement delivers high concentrations of this natural wonder.

Essential Fats There are two essential fatty acids that the body cannot produce and must be obtained from foods. Both are essential for health: Omega 3 Alpha Linolenic Acid and Omega 6 Linoleic Acid. It is important that we get the correct ratio of both fats. We need to add more Omega-3 than Omega-6 into our diet. I use Udo's Oil as it delivers the correct ratios of these important fats. A lack of essential fats can lead to cravings, as the body needs a regular supply of good fats from foods in order to thrive.

Internal Cleanser I take an internal cleanser periodically to cleanse the colon. A lot of unwanted matter resides in the colon and needs to be cleaned out, in order to maintain colon health. I use one that is gentle but effective. Its bases are bioactive, chlorophyll-rich algae, enzymes and herbs.

If you have a specific health challenge or issue there is a wide variety of other supplements that are specific to dealing with them. Some are particularly good for balancing hormones, mood, regulating sleep and enhancing libido, as well as strengthening the immune system. For further advice, contact me on e-mail or my helpline. If you want unprecedented levels of nutritional support, vibrant health, endurance and renewed energy, you need to replace the nutrients lost in cooking and support your best ally against disease – your immune system.

RESOURCES

COURSES RUN BY BERNADETTE

Improve Your Health Naturally: Beginners & Advanced, Dublin Programmes

Join me and learn to make the delicious recipes in this book.

Three-Day Residential Wellness, Cork Programme

Since I began my residential wellness programme thousands of people have come to learn the practical, powerful and effective healing steps of my programme. It is designed to cultivate a healthy lifestyle in a unique and permanent way.

To contact Bernadette
+353(0)1 8452957   Mon–Fri 9-30 a.m. to 5 p.m.
b@changesimply.com
www.changesimply.com
http://www.facebook.com/changesimply
https://twitter.com/bernadettebohan

HIPPOCRATES HEALTH INSTITUTE

1443 Palmdale Court
West Palm Beach, Florida 33411, USA
+1 (561) 471-8876
www.hippocrates.inst.com

REVERSE OSMOSIS AND LIVING WATER SYSTEMS

Renewell Water Ltd.
+353 (0)86 7335874
business@renewellwater.com
www.renewellwater.com

WHEATGRASS & FRESH SPROUTS DELIVERY SERVICES

Christy Stapleton
Kiltegan, Co. Wicklow
+353 (0)59 647346
+353 (0)86 1038605
christystap@gmail.com
https://www.facebook.com/ChristysOrganicWheatgrass

The Happy Pear Living Foods
Leabeg Lower
Newcastle, Co. Wicklow
+353 (0)86 1014181
sprouts@livingfoods.ie
www.livingfoods.ie

THE INSTITUTE OF BIOMAGNETIC THERAPY

www.biomagnetism.ie
www.onehealth.ie
086 811 4073

THERMOMIX POWER BLENDERS

www.thermomixireland.com
www.ukthermomix.com

FURTHER RECOMMENDED READING

Healthful Cuisine, Anna Marie Clement, Healthful Communications, 2006.

Living Foods for Optimum Health, Brian Clement, Prima Health, 1998.

Good Food, John McKenna, Gill & Macmillan, 2013.

What to Eat, Chupi & Luke Sweetman, Gill & Macmillan, 2003.

The Raw Gourmet, Nomi Shannon, Alive Books, 1999.

Hard to Stomach, John McKenna, Gill & Macmillan, 2002.

Immunity Foods for Healthy Kids, Lucy Burney, Duncan Baird, 2004.

Sprouts, Kathleen O'Bannon, Alive Books, 2000.

Juicing – for the Health of It, Siegfried Gursche, Alive Books, 2000.

Juicing for Health, Caroline Wheater, Thorsons, 2001.

Anti-Biotics, John McKenna, Gill & Macmillan 2014.

Chocolate Busters, Jason Vale, Thorsons, 2004.

Fats that Heal, Fats that Kill, Udo Erasmus, Alive Books, 1993.

Cancer: Why We're Still Dying to Know the Truth, Phillip Day, Credence, 1999.

The Plant Programme Jane Plant, J. A., and Gill Tidey, Virgin, 2001.

Fluoride: Drinking Ourselves to Death, Barry Groves, Gill & Macmillan, 2001.

Health Hazards of White Sugar, Lynne Melcombe, Alive Books, 2000.

The Food Doctor, Vicki Edgson & Ian Marber, Collins & Brown, 1999.

Recipes for Self-Healing, David Leggett, Meridian Press, 1999.

Boost Your Immune System Naturally, Beth McEoin, Carlton, 2001.

The Cancer Survivor's Guide, Neal D. Barnard, M. D. Book Publishing Company, 2008.

180 Ways to Effectively Deal with Change, Laurie Caldara, Walk the Talk Company, 2006.

Prevent and Reverse Heart Disease, Caldwell B. Esselstyn, Avery Publishing Group, 2008.

Dr. Dean Ornish Programme for Reversing Heart Disease, Dean Ornish, Ivy Books, 1997.

Encyclopaedia of Natural Healing, Siegfried Gursche, Alive Books, 1997.

The China Study, C. Campbell & T. Campbell, Benbella, 2005.

TO CONTACT BERNADETTE BOHAN

b@changesimply.com
www.changesimply.com

INDEX

vegetables 10
Vitamin D Stuffed Mushrooms 82
vitamins 192
      B vitamins 118, 192
      vitamin C 29, 43, 52, 81
      vitamin D 82, 117, 192
      vitamin E 61, 116

W

Wallner, Renate 78, 101
walnuts
      Amazing Crackers 146
      Delicious Tacos 100
      Dill-iciously Stuffed Peppers 125
      No-sugar, No-cheese-cake 184, **185**
      Not-so-naughty but Nice Pies **186**, 187
      Nuts about Ice Cream 163
      Pizza Time **106**, 107
      Walnut Bonbons 178, **179**
water
      atmospheric 21
      cleansing process and 50
      distillers 19–21
      reverse-osmosis systems 20–1
      tap 19, 27
weight loss 22, 70, 160
Wheat-free Breakfast 66, **67**
wheatgrass 37, 46–7

Y

yeast, nutritional
      Amazing Crackers 146
      Heart-friendly Pesto 140
      Immune-boosting Spinach 131
      No-cheese Parmigiano 91
      Raw-inspiring Lasagne **92**, 93
yoghurt 57
      Dairy-free Yoghurt 60
Yummy Mummy Juice 36
Yutang, Lin 86, 88

Z

Zesty Sprouted Salad 122

ALSO BY BERNADETTE BOHAN

Bernadette Bohan

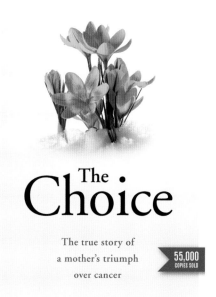

The Choice

The true story of
a mother's triumph
over cancer

55,000 COPIES SOLD

Bernadette Bohan

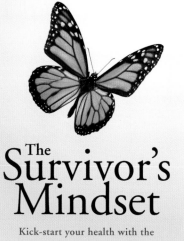

The Survivor's Mindset

Kick-start your health with the
power of your mind and body

The new book from the author of
the bestselling book *The Choice*

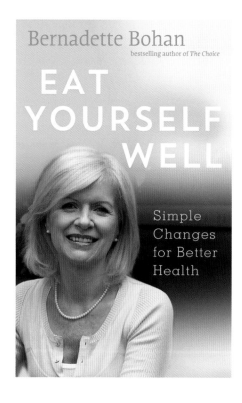

Bernadette Bohan
bestselling author of *The Choice*

EAT YOURSELF WELL

Simple
Changes
for Better
Health